Making the Decision

A Cancer Patient's Guide to Clinical Trials

Making the Decision

A Cancer Patient's Guide to Clinical Trials

Marilyn Mulay
RN, MS, OCN®

University of California at Los Angeles

JONES AND BARTLETT PUBLISHERS
Sudbury, Massachusetts
BOSTON   TORONTO   LONDON   SINGAPORE

World Headquarters
Jones and Bartlett Publishers
40 Tall Pine Drive
Sudbury, MA 01776
978-443-5000
info@jbpub.com
www.jbpub.com

Jones and Bartlett Publishers Canada
2406 Nikanna Road
Mississauga, ON L5C 2W6
CANADA

Jones and Bartlett Publishers International
Barb House, Barb Mews
London W6 7PA
UK

Production Credits

Acquisitions Editor: Penny Glynn
Associate Editor: Thomas Prindle
Production Editor: Jon Workman
Marketing Manager: Taryn Wahlquist
V.P., Manufacturing and Inventory Control:
  Therese Bräuer

Editorial and Production Service:
  Colophon
Composition: Modern Graphics
Printing and Binding: Malloy
  Lithographing
Cover Design: Anne Spencer

Cover Photo Credits

pills: ©1996 PhotoDisc, Inc. All rights reserved. Images provided by ©1996 Tracy Montana/ Photolink; *advisor-technician:* ©1996 PhotoDisc, Inc. All rights reserved. Images provided by ©1996 Tracy Montana/Photolink; *black woman:* ©1997 PhotoDisc, Inc. All rights reserved. Images provided by ©1997 Mel Curtis; *serious boy:* ©1997 PhotoDisc, Inc. All rights reserved. Images provided by ©1997 Mel Curtis; *smiling man 1:* ©1997 PhotoDisc, Inc. All rights reserved. Images provided by ©1997 Mel Curtis; *smiling man 2:* ©1997 PhotoDisc, Inc. All rights reserved. Images provided by ©1997 Mel Curtis.

Library of Congress Cataloging-in-Publication Data
Mulay, Marilyn.
    Making the decision : the cancer patient's guide to clinical trials / by Marilyn Mulay.
      p. cm.
    Includes bibliographical references.
    ISBN 0-7637-1690-1 (pbk.)
      1. Cancer—Treatment—Decision making.   2. Clinical trials—Decision making.   3. Patient education.   I. Title.
    RC270.8 .M85 2001
    616.99′4′0071—dc21   2002041285

Printed in the United States of America
05 04 03 02 01   10 9 8 7 6 5 4 3 2 1

To Monique Dugard Lewis
whose strength sustained her
through treatment, and whose character
and elegance inspired so many
and
to Joseph Mulay
our love and support are with you

*Clinical research offers hope for today
and promise for tomorrow*

Contents

Foreword

The American Cancer Society tells us that, in 2001, more than 1.3 million Americans will be diagnosed with some form of cancer and nearly 560,000 will die from the disease.[1] They go on to tell us that although the percentages of Americans developing and dying of cancer are declining, the absolute number of cases is increasing as a result of an aging population. We have made a great many advances in the treatment of cancers since Richard Nixon declared his "war on cancer" in the 1970s. New therapies have made most testicular cancers and childhood leukemias curable diseases and are now prolonging the lives of many with cancers of the breast, colon, lung, and lymph nodes. But we have room for improvement.

Marilyn Mulay, herself an experienced oncology research nurse and administrator of a large clinical trials program, has written for patients with cancer an excellent reference manual that helps in many ways. For the newly diagnosed patient, it introduces them to the oft-confusing terminology behind many of the factors that health care providers weigh in making treatment recommendations to their patients. For patients with any stage of cancer, it reminds them of the questions they should be asking in deciding where and when to get their treatment. And, above all, it demystifies the world of clinical trials.

The crisis that is cancer exists because we cannot cure everyone diagnosed with the disease. Simply hearing the words, "You have cancer," turns a family's entire world upside down for the fears of suffering, hopelessness, and lack of effective therapies. But researchers are making great strides in understanding what causes and perpetuates cancer and how new therapies can help people live long and active lives with the disease. Only through clinical trials can we continue to make progress in these areas. The fact that fewer than 5% of American cancer patients participate in clinical trials delays this progress significantly.

It is my strong belief that every patient with cancer should educate himself or herself about clinical trial opportunities. Not every patient requires or should receive experimental therapy, but clinical trials also exist to ask patients brief questions about the impact of their disease and treatment on symptoms, lifestyle, workplace, or family. Other trials seek to make the cancer therapy itself more tolerable or safe. But, in all cases, trials seek to improve upon existing treatment in a way that is clear for each potential patient. How to access and interpret information about clinical trials is the focus of this book. It is presented in a manner that is easy to read, no matter how familiar or foreign the world of cancer treatment is. This balanced approach will help patients and caregivers digest the information at their own pace so as to avoid the overload one often feels in a brief visit to the doctor or an overwhelming session on the Internet.

In the oncology community, we have a responsibility to the many patients diagnosed with cancer now and to those who may yet be diagnosed in the years to come. Only by educating our patients about available and appropriate treatments and by the conduct of careful, scientifically sound research can we meet the needs of both groups. Clinical trials are the only way for us to make sure that what we offer our patients today is the best we have to offer and to improve day by day what we might be able to offer our patients in the future.

Lee S. Rosen, M.D.
Director
Cancer Therapy Development Program
University of California at Los Angeles

Reference

1. Greenlee RT, Murray T, Bolden S, *et al.* Cancer Statistics 2001. *CA Cancer J Clin* 2001;51:15–36.

Preface

"You have cancer." This simple sentence forever changes an individual's life. Suddenly, a person is thrust into a world of new places, new people, and a language that seems foreign. The healthy individual assumes the role of a patient and is asked to make decisions based on a flood of new and, often, poorly understood information. The decisions frequently have life-altering consequences. At the same time, the new patient is dealing with the emotional upheaval caused by the cancer diagnosis. A multitude of questions and concerns about health, finances, and the future often take over the conscious mind, interfering with the individual's normal ability to make rational decisions.

In an effort to become informed, patients often visit the Internet. However, sorting through all of the information found there to determine what applies to this specific situation can be very difficult. Family and friends, and friends of friends, feel compelled to tell the new patient stories about other people who "have exactly what you have." These tales often border on the worse horror stories ever heard.

As soon as the diagnosis is confirmed, the primary care physician typically refers the patient to a surgeon or medical oncologist to begin treatment. Without time to establish a trusting relationship, the new physician typically begins to recommend treatment options. The patient, with no experience in the medical arena and little information, really is incapable of making an informed decision and, therefore, may accept the physician's recommendation on blind faith. So much information is given in such a short period of time, that it is impossible for the patient to process and use it effectively. Patients' decisions often are driven by the idea that cancer must be treated *immediately.* A sense of urgency can rush the patient into a treatment that may not be the best available option.

Patients need to understand that cancer is a term that encompasses more than 100 different diseases. Therefore, the treatment of cancer requires many different approaches. These treatments may be surgery, radiation, chemotherapy, or a combination of modalities. The body of knowledge about cancer treatment is based on an understanding of the specific disease and its typical behavior. However, the treatment of cancer is determined not only by the disease but also on how it manifests itself in a particular person. Moreover, treatment is not a one-time decision, but rather a complex, ongoing process. Individuals most likely will be asked to make many decisions along the continuum of their care. Their stage of life, responsibilities, financial situation, and value system all impact the decisions.

The medical community's understanding about cancer treatments is an evolving process. Research into how cancer grows and how to stop it is ongoing. New approaches to treatment are continually being tested, and patient participation in research through clinical trials is necessary to advance knowledge about treatments. However, a recent study indicated that 85% of patients were not aware of clinical trials. Many physicians also are not well informed about the availability of clinical trials or simply assume that their patients are not eligible. Therefore, patients must often be their own advocates.

Unfortunately, lack of patient participation in cancer clinical trials delays the gathering of information that could lead to medical breakthroughs. For example, in breast cancer, radical mastectomy procedures were proven in clinical trials to be no more effective than lumpectomy plus radiation. This finding saved many women from radical surgery.

This book is designed to give patients the basic information necessary to become informed consumers about treatment decisions. Medical terminology is simplified to understandable terms and standard treatments are explained to form a solid foundation for the process of decision-making. Understanding many of the components impacting treatment decisions puts the patients in a better position to make good choices.

The book begins by discussing *The Cancer Problem,* its risk factors, and basic pathology in Chapter 1. Chapter 2, *Defining the Disease,* is designed to help patients through the process of biopsy and diagnosis and then to understand the diagnosis. What is a pathology report and what does it really say? In Chapter 3, typical treatment options are discussed. Because cancer is so many different diseases, discussion of specific treatments in this book is not possible. The information provided here is designed to help the patient understand the various treatment types and to define the structure of *Treatment Decision-Making*.

For many of the common cancers, such as breast, lung, and colon cancer, there are well-known standard therapies. However, there is still a great need for improvement in treatments that will positively impact both survival and the patient's quality of life. Further, for some rare cancers, there are no treatment options that have proven to be effective. New drugs and therapies must be developed, but the process of drug development and testing in both animals and humans is lengthy and arduous. Defining new therapies is an ongoing quest of testing new procedures, experimental drugs, and combinations of approved and experimental drugs. The testing of the experimental therapies in humans is called clinical trials. Chapter 4 describes the process of *Drug Development* and Chapter 5 defines the various types and phases of *Clinical Trials*.

The future of cancer therapy depends on the results of clinical trials. Useful information is dependent on patient participation, but currently only 3% of cancer care is given in clinical trials. Patients often fear that they will not be told the truth about the testing. There are concerns that they may receive a placebo (sugar pill) or be used as a guinea pig. However, there are many regulatory agencies and laws in place to protect the patients from unethical practices. Chapter 6, *The Business of Clinical Research*, outlines the process of taking a drug from the laboratory to the treatment facility to begin human testing. Chapter 7 gives the history of the development of safeguards and discusses *The Patient's Rights*, particularly through the process of informed consent.

Hundreds of clinical trials are being conducted all over the world. Chapter 8, *How to Find a Clinical Trial*, assists patients who are interested in participating in clinical trials to find trials and determine their eligibility. Once an appropriate trial has been found and eligibility has been established, the patient must also consider the costs of participating in a clinical trial. In a pharmaceutical study, the pharmaceutical company pays many of the costs involved in the trial, but other costs are billed to the patient's insurance company. In the world of managed care, referrals and authorizations have become a complex issue. If a patient chooses to participate in a trial that is located away from his or her home, living expenses are also a major concern. Chapter 9, *Understanding the Finances*, discusses many of these issues.

When all of the concerns have been addressed successfully, a patient is enrolled in a clinical trial. The patient's role in data collection is an important part of the study. Chapter 10, *Care of the Research Subject,* explains what a patient can expect during the trial and how to assist the investigators to provide optimal care and collect useful information.

Chapter 11, *Making the Decision,* gathers together all of the information and walks the patient through the process of deciding if and when participation in a clinical trial is the appropriate decision. The patient's disease, its stage, prior therapies, and the availability of appropriate trials all are part of the decision, and each decision is specific to the patient and his or her current situation. Therefore, this information may be useful at various times during the course of the patient's treatment.

Recent research suggests that patient education and a complete informed consent process may overcome the lack of patient participation in clinical trials. This book is designed to meet that need. Armed with the information contained in this book, a patient will be better prepared to make well-informed decisions about cancer treatment in general and in the context of clinical trials in particular.

Acknowledgments

Many, many thanks to:

All of the patients who encouraged me to write this book and continued to give support throughout the process.

Dr. Lee Rosen and Joseph Brown for their professional support and personal belief in me.

Those who, in addition to their support, helped to define the content of this book and provided editorial assistance: Mandy Parson, Kelli Petersen, Don Friedman; the editorial staff at Jones and Bartlett, in particular Penny Glynn, Christine Tridente, and Thomas Prindle; and the production staff at Colophon, in particular, Peg Latham.

My family, Dana and Gus Lira, and James, Trisha, and Samuel Rudnick for your love, encouragement, and support.

You cannot hold a torch to light another's path without brightening your own.

Anonymous

CHAPTER 1

The Cancer Problem

▮ What Is Cancer?

More than 100 different diseases are called cancer. Cancers are classified into two general categories: hematologic malignancies and solid tumor malignancies. **Hematologic malignancies,** such as leukemia and multiple myeloma, are diseases that occur as a result of an abnormality in a certain type of blood cell. Lymphoma, also considered a hematologic malignancy, is an abnormality in the lymph system of the body. **Solid tumor malignancies** are diseases, such as breast, lung, prostate, and colorectal cancer, in which an abnormal, discrete mass of cells, called a *tumor,* is present. The common element is that, in each disease, abnormal cells grow and spread in an uncontrolled manner. In a healthy adult, normal cells have a natural protective mechanism that limits their growth and defines a specified life cycle. In cancer, the normal process is disrupted.

Cancer is the second leading cause of death in the United States, affecting one in three Americans. Each year, more than one million new cases of cancer are diagnosed and more than 500,000 Americans die of the disease. However, cancer is no longer the death sentence that so many associate with the diagnosis. Approximately 8.4 million Americans alive today are cancer survivors (1). Some of these people are considered cured, others are in remission, and others still have some evidence of disease.

■ Why Does Cancer Happen?

Often, the first question asked is, "How did I get this?" In most cases, the actual cause of the disease is unknown. Observations show that lifestyle and lifestyle-related behaviors are most likely to cause or promote the development of cancer (2). Cancer research has helped identify some occupational and environmental factors that are implicated in the development of cancer. Some of these factors are controllable; others are not.

Uncontrollable Internal Factors

Cancer starts with a mutation of an individual's gene, the body's chemical control board. Some of these mutations are hereditary, particularly in certain cancers, such as some breast and colon cancers. The knowledge that a first-degree family member (mother, father, sister, brother, or grandparent) may have passed on a mutated gene should heighten an individual's alertness to screening, typically done more frequently or beginning at an earlier age than the rest of the population. Only about 5% to 10% of cancers are hereditary. The rest of the cancers are believed to be caused by controllable factors (1).

Controllable Factors

Tobacco use, which accounts for 30% of all cancer deaths each year, is probably the most avoidable behavior. Cancers of the lung, mouth, pharynx, larynx, esophagus, pancreas, uterine cervix, kidney, and bladder are all associated with tobacco. In 87% of lung cancers, tobacco is implicated (1).

Cigarette smoking accounts for thousands of deaths each year. In 1995, it was reported that, in developed countries, approximately 2.1 million people died of smoking-related diseases (3). However, in cancer, cigarette smoking is not the sole culprit. Cigars contain many of the same carcinogens as cigarettes. In addition, smokeless tobacco has been falsely believed to be harmless. In fact, most of the same carcinogens that are in cigarettes also are found in other forms of tobacco. Risks of dying from cancer caused by tobacco use are several times higher when compared to nonsmokers (1).

Second-hand smoke is implicated in lung cancer. Approximately 3,000 nonsmoking adults die each year as a result of second-hand smoke. The known carcinogens, benzene, 2-naphthylamine, 4-amino-biphenyl, and polonium-210, are all in second-hand smoke, along with at least ten more chemicals that probably are carcinogens (1).

Scientific evidence shows that approximately one-third of cancer deaths are related to nutrition and other lifestyle factors. High-fat diets are implicated in several cancers, including breast and colorectal cancers. About 3% of all cancer deaths can be attributed to alcohol. Use of both alcohol and tobacco has a negative, synergistic effect on many cancers (4).

Skin cancer accounts for 1.3 million cases of cancer each year. Many could be prevented by appropriate use of protection from the sun, especially during childhood (1).

No one knows exactly if or when a certain lifestyle choice will cause cancer to occur. However, it is believed that controlling weight, exercising, eating a well-balanced diet, and avoiding behaviors such as excess alcohol consumption and tobacco use will help prevent the disease.

Common sense should be the guide. For example, the media may report the results of a study about a cancer-causing agent. It is important to look beyond the promotional clips and not just read the headlines; look at the study methods and how the conclusion is reached. Recognize that the amount of a substance that is fed to the animals may be many times more than any normal adult would consume in a lifetime. Also, just as the researchers have been quite successful in curing cancer in mice, the translation of those results to humans is not always possible. The same premise is true of these types of studies; the behavior studied in mice may not produce the same results in humans.

Uncontrollable External Factors

Environmental factors, such as chemicals, radiation, and viruses, have been implicated in the development of cancer, although current estimates indicate that only 5% of all cancers can be traced to these sources (2). Assessment of the safe amount of exposure to these substances is difficult to achieve.

By conducting studies in the workplace, certain carcinogens have been identified. In the studies, some employees who have been in sustained contact with high levels of certain chemicals demonstrate higher incidences of specific cancers. It also has been found that the duration of exposure is an important part of the equation: the longer the exposure, the greater the risk of disease. In some cases, simultaneous exposures, for example, asbestos and cigarette smoke, can greatly increase risks (1).

Concerns about radiation exposure from holes in the ozone layer, dental or medical radiographic studies, and radon have received a great deal of media attention. However, only high-frequency radiation (i.e., ionizing and ultraviolet radiation) has been implicated in causing cancer.

Simple precautions make good sense. As discussed earlier, careful use of sunscreen products provide protection against ultraviolet radiation. Similarly, commercial products are available to test homes for radon, which has been implicated in lung cancer. Exposure to radon combined with cigarette smoke increases the risk.

Although concerns about radiation exposure from x-rays have been raised, it is foolish to sacrifice x-ray studies needed for medical or dental health for fear of radiation exposure. New technology has minimized the amount of exposure from x-rays to very safe levels. Again, common sense must prevail.

In addition, concerns about pesticides, toxic waste, and nuclear power plant emissions all add to the fear of developing cancer. There is no definitive proof that any of these exposures actually causes cancer. Overall, controllable factors probably have a higher impact on the development of cancer than uncontrollable factors.

■ How Does Cancer Happen?

The most commonly accepted theory is that cancer occurs in several phases:

- Initiation
- Promotion
- Progression

Normal cells duplicate themselves through a series of chemical events in which deoxyribonucleic acid (DNA, the genetic material in the cell) is able to divide and create exact replicas of the gene-containing strands. In cancer, the DNA is damaged by either a genetic mutation or a **carcinogen** (as discussed earlier).

This first stage is known as **initiation,** a mistake that occurs in the transcription of a gene. A damaged cell may repair itself or remain permanently changed without consequence of cancer. However, if the cell remains damaged, it is susceptible to develop cancer if it encounters a promoter.

Promotion, the second stage, is a process by which carcinogens are introduced into the cell. If a cell that has already encountered an initiator then comes in contact with a promoter, a succession of events begins that allows the cell to defy its natural life cycle, grow uncontrollably, and become immortal. If the immune system of an individual (host) cannot halt the mutated cell, then the damaged cell replicates millions of times, forming a mass of abnormal cells. When the mass achieves a size of at least 1 cm, it can be detected by either palpation (it can be felt) or radiographic examination. It may take years for the mass to develop to a size that can be seen or felt. The official diagnosis of cancer is made only after cells from the mass are retrieved, viewed under a microscope by a pathologist, and determined to be cancerous (2). If the development of cancer stopped at the promotion phase, most cancers could be removed and would have little more effect on the host than the common cold.

Unfortunately, many cancers are not detected before the last phase, **progression.** During this phase, the cancer spreads from its original location by either **invasion** or **metastasis.** Invasion occurs when the cancer grows into surrounding tissue, for example, into lymph nodes close to the primary cancer. This is known as **regional spread.** Sometimes, the cancer cells will travel via the circulatory system (blood) to distant sites, for example, a lung cancer that spreads to the liver. This is known as **distant metastasis.**

Although every cancer patient would like to know how cancer got into his or her body, the fact is that there may never be a definitive answer. If there is a familial tendency or predisposition, it is important for family members to be proactive about screening procedures and to eliminate unhealthy habits. For the patient diagnosed with cancer, energy must be placed into understanding treatment options and making informed decisions.

■ References

1. *Cancer facts & figures 2000.* Atlanta, GA: American Cancer Society, 2000: 1–3,15,28–30.
2. Mulay M. *Step-by-step guide to clinical trials.* Sudbury, MA: Jones and Bartlett, 2001.
3. Centers for Disease Control and Prevention. Cigarette smoking-attributable mortality and years of potential life lost—United States, 1984. *MMWR* 1997; 46:444–450.
4. Groenwald S, Frogge M, Goodman M, et al. *Cancer nursing: principles and practice.* Sudbury, MA: Jones and Bartlett, 1997.

CHAPTER 2

Defining the Disease

■ Understanding the Pathology Report

Before a definitive diagnosis of cancer can be made, cells must be retrieved from the suspicious mass in solid tumor malignancies or from the bone marrow in hematologic malignancies and examined under a microscope by a pathologist. Specimens for biopsy are obtained in two ways, surgically or by aspiration.

Bone Marrow Biopsy

In hematologic malignancies, an abnormality noted on a simple blood test called a *complete blood count (CBC)* may alert a physician to a serious problem. In order to obtain cells for diagnosis, a bone marrow biopsy must be done. Bone marrow is located in the pelvic bones, the femurs in the upper leg, and the sternum or breastbone. The biopsy is obtained by placing a large needle into the bone marrow and extracting (or aspirating) cells via a syringe. Most often, the biopsy is done on an outpatient basis and the cells are taken from the pelvic bone. The patient may be given medications to cause relaxation and reduce discomfort. The cells are placed on glass slides and sent to the pathologist for analysis.

Fine Needle Aspiration

If there is a mass that can be palpated or felt, such as a lump in the neck or breast, some physicians opt for a **fine needle aspiration (FNA)** as a means of collecting cells to define the nature of the lump. The area is anesthetized with a numbing solution and cells or fluid is withdrawn through a needle that has been placed into the mass. The resulting specimen is called an **aspirate.** The pathologist looks for abnormal cells under the microscope to determine if the mass is benign or malignant.

FNA can be done in the office with minimal time and discomfort for the patient; however, there is potential for problems with the procedure. If the mass is small or not easily accessible, the needle may pass through the mass or be placed to the side of it. If the cells are retrieved from surrounding normal tissue rather than from the suspicious mass, a false-negative report can result. Sometimes, cells may be damaged in the process or an aspirate may only indicate that the fluid is suspicious for malignancy. In that case, a surgical biopsy still must be done for a definitive diagnosis. If possible, it is preferable to do a less invasive procedure first.

If the suspicious mass is not amenable to FNA, a surgical biopsy may be done. The procedure is more involved because it requires an incision in the skin. Whenever the body's integrity is invaded (the skin is opened), care must be taken to avoid infection; therefore, a surgical biopsy often is done in the operating room. Typically, the patient remains in a recovery area for a couple of hours after the procedure to ensure that no bleeding or reaction occurs.

Surgical Biopsy

Surgical biopsies fall into two categories: incisional and excisional. An **incisional biopsy** is used to remove a piece of a mass when the mass is large and not amenable to complete removal. For example, patients with lymphoma may present with a large mass in the chest. Because the entire mass cannot be removed surgically, an incisional biopsy is done to confirm the diagnosis. Once the exact diagnosis is known, further treatment decisions are made.

When the mass is small and discrete, an **excisional biopsy,** removal of the entire mass, is done. For example, an entire lymph node may be removed for pathologic analysis. When possible, this is the preferable means for biopsy because the entire mass can be examined. This eliminates the possibility of a specimen that is nondiagnostic because of damage to the cells or an insufficient number of cells for analysis.

Tumor Block

Tissue taken from the biopsy is embedded in paraffin wax. This **tumor block** is stored in the pathology department of the hospital where the surgery was done. Pieces of the block are sliced off and placed on glass slides to be viewed under the microscope for analysis. For certain treatments, a patient may be asked to contact the pathology laboratory to obtain a slice of the tumor block for testing to determine if the tumor expresses some feature that responds to a new therapy. At that time, the laboratory will remove a thin slice of the original tumor sent in for analysis. It is very important not to have the entire block sent because it could be lost or misplaced.

Patients whose diagnosis was made by bone marrow biopsy or FNA will not have a tumor block. An aspirate is a liquid that cannot be embedded in paraffin. Rather, those cells are placed on slides that also are maintained in the pathology department.

■ Pathology Report

In the event of leukemia, the pathology report will identify the type as either

- Chronic or acute
- Myelogenous, lymphocytic, or promyelocytic

The results of additional testing of the cells identify subtypes and the chromosomal analysis. All of the information is important in determining treatment.

If the diagnosis is multiple myeloma, the disease is defined by cell type: IgA, IgG, IgM, or IgE (immunoglobulin). The patient's urine is analyzed for an abnormality called a kappa light chain. All of this information classifies the disease into a specific type and dictates the treatment options.

With solid tumors and lymphoma, a pathology report can define the biologic behavior and the tissue of origin of the cancer. The behavior is defined as either **benign** or **malignant.** In solid tumors, there are a variety of different types of malignant tumors arising from different tissues. The most common types are

- Sarcoma, from connective tissue similar to that found in ligaments
- Carcinoma, from epithelial tissue such as that found in skin

Carcinomas are divided further by the cell type of epithelial tissue:

- Adenocarcinoma, from epithelial tissue similar to that found in glands
- Squamous, from epithelial tissue such as that lining the mouth

These distinctions are important in identifying the appropriate treatment for a particular cancer. Cancers arising from connective tissues behave differently than those arising from glandular epithelial tissue. Treatment options are defined by the type of cells that form the disease.

The pathology report also gives details about differentiation of the cells. Cell differentiation refers to the degree of difference from a normal cell appearance and can vary from well differentiated to poorly differentiated. Well-differentiated cancer cells look more like normal cells than poorly differentiated cells. Cancers with poorly differentiated cells typically have a poorer prognosis than those with better differentiation.

For some diagnoses, additional tests, such as stains and hormone or receptor tests, may be done on tumor cells. The information gleaned from special testing helps to further define the disease. If there is any doubt about the diagnosis based on the biopsy, the slides may be sent for further analysis to another institution that has more experience in reading pathology slides. If surgery is indicated, additional tissue will be sent for pathologic analysis after removal of the tumor. Sometimes, a larger specimen will clarify a diagnosis. A definitive diagnosis is extremely important because it dictates treatment decisions. Treatment for different diagnoses varies significantly.

Findings in the pathology report are only a means of defining a diagnosis. Further testing, such as computerized tomography (CT) scans, usually is needed to define the full extent of the disease.

■ Bronchial Brushings

In certain types of lung cancer or disease that has spread to the lung, no discrete mass is visible. Instead, the lining of the lungs may be thickened. In this case, it may not be possible to obtain tissue or aspirate. Often, **bronchoscopy** (a procedure in which a lighted tube is threaded through the mouth into the respiratory tract) is done to visualize the site. A brush is inserted through the tube, and cells are obtained for a pathologist to examine. The cells from the brushings are placed on slides to be viewed under the microscope. Again in this situation, no tumor block can be made.

■ Radiographic Staging

Once a malignancy is identified, radiographic studies, such as CT, magnetic resonance imaging (MRI), and/or bone scans, are ordered to determine if the disease is contained at the primary site **(localized)** or whether it has spread either locally **(regional spread)** or to distant sites **(metastasized).** An irregularity seen on a scan may be presumed to be metastatic disease, but without a biopsy, it is only a presumption.

Radiologists who are experienced in reading oncology scans may be able to distinguish metastatic lesions from scarring or other disease processes. However, in some cases, more sophisticated radiographic examinations, such as positron emission tomography (PET) scans or MRIs using special contrast mediums, may help to clarify the findings. At other times, another biopsy may be recommended to confirm the diagnosis of metastatic disease, or a questionable lesion can be biopsied during the primary surgery.

Technology has become very refined. There are a variety of radiology studies available to help define a disease. The physician together with the radiologist is the best source to determine what studies are necessary to obtain the most useful information. Disease in certain areas of the body is best seen by specific studies. For example, soft tissue is visualized best by MRI rather than CT scan. Although bone lesions may be seen on CT scan, they are best defined by bone scan.

Contrast agents or radioactive isotopes sometimes are given to ensure that the images on CT scan clearly define any irregularity. For example, before CT of the abdomen, the patient drinks a contrast liquid to help distinguish the stomach and bowel from other structures in the body. Intravenous contrast before chest CTs will give a more distinct picture to best define abnormalities. Many contrast agents are iodine based, so if a patient is allergic to iodine or shellfish, it is very important to communicate this information to the radiologist.

■ Surgical Staging

Surgery remains the patient's best option for a cure from cancer. During surgery, the surgeon not only resects (removes) the primary tumor, but also feels or palpates surrounding lymph nodes and looks at the entire surgical field. Direct visualization and palpation are the best means to determine the full extent of the disease. Tumors that are accessible are removed. Regional lymph nodes typically are removed for analysis as well. All excised tissue is sent to the laboratory for pathologic examination. Another pathology report then is issued, listing the diagnosis for each specimen (piece of tissue) received.

▉ TNM Classification

The TNM system is a system used by the medical community to define disease, as follows:

T = tumor
N = node
M = metastasis

Not every cancer will have a TNM classification assigned. For example, defining the tumor in a cancer of unknown primary origin is not possible. A report containing a Tx, Nx, or Mx indicates there was insufficient information to assess the extent of disease. The exact definition of each category varies by type of cancer. For purposes of illustration, the system is applied here to colon cancer.

Think of the colon as a tube. Figure 2-1 is a depiction of the colon sliced open to visualize the inner layers. The mucosa is the innermost layer. The submucosa and serosa make up the next two layers. The muscle layer is the outermost layer, with the outer rim creating the bowel wall

T Categories

- *Tis* is a tumor *in situ*, meaning the tumor has not grown beyond the inner layer of the colon, the mucosa. This is the earliest stage of cancer, when the cancerous cells remain confined to the tissue of origin.
- *T1* indicates the cancer has grown through the mucosa and into submucosa.

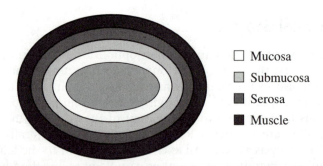

☐ Mucosa
▨ Submucosa
▦ Serosa
▉ Muscle

Figure 2-1 Layers of the colon

- *T2* indicates the cancerous cells have grown into the muscle layer.
- *T3* indicates the cancer has grown into the subserosa.
- *T4* indicates the cancer has grown completely through the wall of the colon and into nearby tissues or organs.

N Categories

- *N0* indicates there is no lymph node involvement.
- *N1* indicates that one to three lymph nodes in the region of the primary tumor contain cancer.
- *N2* indicates there are four or more cancerous regional lymph nodes.

M Categories

- *M0* indicates there is no evidence of distant spread of the disease.
- *M1* indicates there is distant spread of disease.

■ Assigning the Stage of Disease

Many different **staging** systems have been developed over the years. Recently, staging systems have been simplified to define the extent of disease by stages from 0 to IV. Although the staging varies somewhat by disease, the basic premises are the same. The following explanation again uses colon cancer for purposes of illustration.

Cancer in its earliest stage is called **stage 0** or **tumor *in situ* (Tis).** For example, a cancerous polyp is seen during colonoscopy. If the disease is confined to the tip of the polyp, it can be snared and removed during the colonoscopy (Fig. 2-2). The tumor then is examined by a

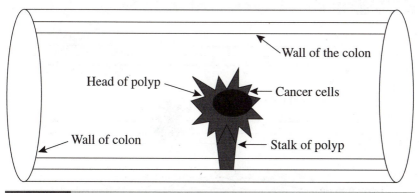

Figure 2-2 Stage 0 colon cancer. Tis, N0, M0

pathologist to ensure that the cells on the edge of the specimen are normal. Clear margins indicate that all of the cancer was removed. An annual colonoscopy is generally recommended to monitor for recurrence.

Stage I disease is early-stage disease that can be cured with surgery. In the case of a mushroom-shaped polyp (pedunculated) where the cancer has spread to the stalk or a flat polyp (sessile) that has invaded the wall, more extensive surgery is needed to ensure that all cancerous cells are removed (Fig. 2-3). Typically, a surgeon will choose to remove the involved section of the bowel. At the time of surgery, the surrounding area and lymph nodes can be visualized and palpated to ensure that the cancer is confined.

In stages 0 and I, most patients will have a section of the tumor removed by either colonoscopy or laparoscopy (through a tube inserted into the abdominal wall). Postoperative recovery typically is uncomplicated, and the patient returns to a normal lifestyle with instructions for annual or semiannual follow-up visits.

Stage II cancer typically is defined as cancer that has penetrated deeper into tissue and, in fact, through the bowel wall, but not into surrounding organs or tissue (Fig. 2-4).

In stage II colon cancer, a surgical cure is the expected outcome.

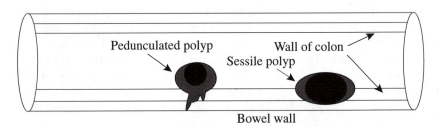

Figure 2-3 Stage I colon cancer. T1, N0, M0. T2, N0, M0

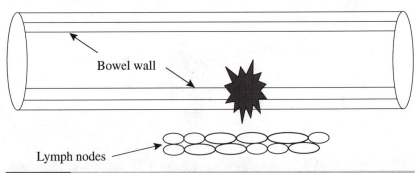

Figure 2-4 Stage II colon cancer. T3, N0, M0. T4, N0, M0

Assuming that nothing unexpected is seen during the surgery (spread of disease is too small to be seen on preoperative scans), all of the disease will be removed. Understand that the surgically removed tumor will again be sent to the pathologist for analysis; a larger piece of the tumor may yield more information. Also, the excised tumor is examined for clear margins to ensure all of the tumor has been removed. Follow-up is dictated by the stage of disease and the postoperative surgical pathology report.

Stage III colon cancer presents a new set of problems because the cancer, regardless of the penetration of the tumor into the bowel wall, has infiltrated local (regional) lymph nodes (Fig. 2-5). Recall that N1 represents infiltration of one to three lymph nodes; N2 represents four or more.

Most colon cancers involving regional lymph nodes can be surgically resected. Recall that treatment decisions are based on the depth of penetration of the tumor as well as lymph node involvement. For example, all stage III colon cancers will be treated with chemotherapy because there is an increased risk of **micrometastasis,** cells that have traveled away from the primary site but are too small to be seen on CT scan. Use of chemotherapy in this setting is called **adjuvant therapy,** treatment when all known cancer cells have been surgically removed. Although chemotherapy is always given for stage III colon cancer, opinions differ about the use of adjuvant chemotherapy for stage II colon cancer and sometimes are dependent on the differentiation of the tumor.

Stage IV cancer is defined by disease that has spread to distant sites. For example, a patient may have a cancerous tumor in the colon that is resected. However, more tumors are found in the liver, a site far from the cancer's origin. Known as distant metastases, all patients with stage IV disease must have systemic chemotherapy. Even if the metastasis is amenable to surgical removal, it must be presumed that if the disease traveled to the liver, it also may have traveled elsewhere but possibly is not visible to the surgeon or on CT scan.

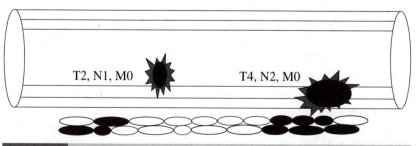

T2, N1, M0   T4, N2, M0

Figure 2-5 Stage III colon cancer. Any T, N1, M0. Any T, N2, M0

■ Presumptive Diagnoses

Sometimes, a biopsy report will read *metastatic adenocarcinoma, unknown primary.* Despite review of the pathology slides and an extensive workup, including mammograms, colonoscopy, and CT scans, a definitive diagnosis cannot be made. Occasionally, an elevated tumor marker may suggest a particular origin, but it cannot be confirmed. Cases such as this often are presented at physicians' conferences to gather collective expertise. Typically, when a confirmed diagnosis is not possible, a presumptive diagnosis is made.

■ Case Study

Betty Cole presented to her primary care physician with a lump in her neck. She was referred to a surgeon who performed an FNA in his office. The resulting pathology report read *metastatic adenocarcinoma, unknown primary.* The pathology slides were sent to the university hospital to be read by the pathologist, but the diagnosis came back the same.

Initial blood work did not reveal any abnormalities. CT scans of the chest, abdomen, and pelvis were all normal. In looking at the most common organ systems that produce adenocarcinoma, Betty had a mammogram; the result was normal. Her pelvic examination did not reveal anything abnormal, and her Pap smear was negative. Upper endoscopy and colonoscopy showed no abnormalities. Thinking that a positive bone scan might narrow the search to those diseases that often metastasize to the bones, a bone scan was done but the result was normal. Looking at diseases that often are insidious because they are not well visualized in radiographic studies, tumor markers were drawn for ovarian and pancreatic cancer.

The level of pancreatic tumor marker CA19-9 was significantly elevated. Yet another look at the abdomen failed to demonstrate a physical manifestation of tumor. To obtain a piece of pancreatic tissue for biopsy would have required major surgery that would have delayed therapy for several weeks to allow for recovery. The presumptive diagnosis of pancreatic cancer was made and treatment was begun.

If a definitive diagnosis is not possible, physicians call upon their experience and expertise to define the disease using the available information. It is important to begin therapy without wasting valuable time looking for the elusive tumor. Sometimes, the patient's response to therapy will help to confirm the diagnosis.

■ Tumor Markers

Some tumor cells release a chemical into the blood stream that can be measured by a special blood test. Some **tumor markers** are very specific for a particular cancer, such as prostate-specific antigen (PSA) in prostate cancer. An elevated PSA level is a good indicator that prostate cancer is present and often is used as a means to follow disease progression.

Other tumor markers are not specific for a particular cancer and are not as sensitive indicators. For example, carcinoembryonic antigen (CEA) can be found in breast cancer, lung cancer, and several gastrointestinal cancers, such as colon, gastric, and esophageal cancer. Smokers have a higher CEA level than nonsmokers. Patients can have very little disease seen on CT scans but have a high CEA level. On the other hand, a low CEA level may be present in a patient with a large tumor burden. Typically, if the CEA level is elevated at initial diagnosis, it likely will be helpful to follow the course of the disease.

> ### Important Note:
>
> Treatment decisions should not be based on tumor markers alone. Monthly blood tests to monitor tumor markers are a relatively inexpensive and noninvasive means to monitor disease status. An elevation may suggest radiographic testing to further evaluate the current extent of the disease.

Table 2-1 lists some tumor markers that are used for specific cancers.

Table 2-1 Common Tumor Markers	
Tumor Marker	**Cancer**
CA27-29	Breast
β-HCG, α-FP	Testicular
CEA	Breast, colorectal, esophageal, lung, gastric
CA19-9	Pancreatic
Thyroglobulin, calcitonin	Thyroid
CA125	Ovarian
PSA	Prostate

■ Reference

1. Weisburger JH, Williams GM. Causes of cancer. In: Murphy GP, Lawrence W, Jr., Lenhard RE, Jr., eds. *American Cancer Society Textbook of Clinical Oncology,* 2nd ed. Washington, DC: Pan American Health Organization, Publications Marketing Program, 1995:10–39.

CHAPTER 3

Treatment Decision-Making

An individual diagnosed with cancer is thrust from the role of healthy person to that of a patient with cancer. Many concerns about job, family, independence, finances, and the future crowd into his or her conscious mind. At the same time, there is a multitude of decisions facing the patient, from selecting doctors to choosing treatments. A patient may feel overwhelmed and even incapable of making any decision. Although timely treatment is important, patients must be sure to take enough time to understand all options and make sound decisions.

The process of decision-making is the same as that for other decisions made by individuals in their lives: gather information, define the options, evaluate the choices, and make the best possible choice. Remember that evaluation is often the most important part of the process, and most decisions can be altered if the outcome is not what was expected.

The patient's value system is an important consideration in treatment decisions. Some patients believe every effort must be made to fight the disease, and no hardship is too much to endure. For other individuals, the financial and/or physical sacrifices are not worth the potential outcome. Many of these decisions are based on the extent of the disease at a specific time and other considerations, such as family and finances. Decisions vary from patient to patient and from situation to situation. A patient's value system will drive the decision-making process.

■ Seeking a Second Opinion

Patients often are confused about the need for a second opinion. They wonder how, when, and where to get one. Sometimes they worry that the primary physician will feel slighted if they seek another opinion. Considering the importance of the diagnosis and the ramifications of correct decisions and appropriate treatment, one cannot overstate the need to seek the best available advice following a diagnosis of cancer. Getting more than one opinion can be very helpful because the patient gathers additional information and, potentially, other points of view.

People often believe that treatment must start immediately upon the diagnosis of cancer. This is rarely the case. If a patient has a condition that is life-threatening, for example, a bowel obstruction, then immediate surgery is necessary. However, in most cases, an individual with a newly-diagnosed cancer can and should take the time to see another oncologist to ensure that all possible options have been presented.

Patients may turn to their primary physician or local oncologist for recommendations on the latest approved therapies for each cancer diagnosis. However, it is nearly impossible for physicians to stay abreast of all of the clinical trials being conducted all over the country. Many oncologists will assist the patient to arrange a second consultation. Every physician should be able to provide the name of the nearest Comprehensive Cancer Center.

The National Cancer Institute (NCI), which is part of the National Institutes of Health (NIH), oversees Comprehensive Cancer Centers throughout the United States. At these centers, a patient has access to information on where the latest treatments are being tested and utilized. Most centers have a physician referral line where a patient will be directed to the appropriate department and physician. Academic medical centers are excellent sources for second opinions. Call the universities in the local area for information about their cancer programs. The Internet offers a wealth of information about cancer in general and specifically about different diagnoses and cancer treatments (see Chapter 8 for more information on this finding in clinical trials).

Most Comprehensive Cancer Centers and academic medical centers maintain web sites that provide current information about the center and current clinical trials. If patients are unfamiliar with the Internet, friends, neighbors (especially teenagers), or local librarians may be able to help.

Other people with cancer can be excellent resources to locate treatment centers. The Wellness Community and similar organizations have centers in many major cities and can help connect individuals to treatment centers.

Seeking a second opinion at a major medical center does not require that the patient receive treatment at that facility. Often, the recommendation will be for standard therapy that can be given at a community oncologist's office.

Whereas a second opinion often is useful, third and fourth opinions usually are excessive and only lead to confusion. If the second option differs from the original recommendation, the physicians often confer to define the best option. If the first two consultations result in completely opposing opinions, then another consultation may help. However, some patients will keep shopping for an oncologist until they find one who will tell them what they want to hear. Delaying treatment for 2 to 3 weeks to gather information is acceptable. When the process drags on for 2 to 3 months, the patient should be encouraged to make a decision and proceed with treatment.

■ A Word of Caution

Some people find a newly diagnosed individual a receptive source to tell horror stories. Beware of those who tell stories about their sister-in-law's cousin who has exactly what the patient has and who was grossly misdiagnosed and mistreated. Stories like these, told third and fourth hand by well-meaning, but misinformed, people, often are filled with incorrect information and create unfounded fears and worries. The patient's physician is the best source of information.

■ The Patient's Role in the Consultation

In order to get the best result from the consultation, the physician needs as much information as possible. It is essential that the patient bring the following documents to the visit:

- Pathology report and slides
- Laboratory reports
- Computerized tomography (CT) scan reports and films (if applicable)
- Past medical history

- Operative reports (if applicable)
- Treatment history
- List of current medications

It is preferable to bring *copies* of all of these records so they can be retained at the consulting institution. Always keep the originals for the patient's own records.

When registering for a new patient appointment, the patient may be asked to complete a patient questionnaire containing specific questions about his or her past and current state of health. Be sure to advise the medical personnel about any allergies the patient may have. If all of the documents noted above are available, completing the questionnaire should be easy.

Typically, the consulting physician, or one of his or her staff, will review the records before the patient is brought to an examination room. At a teaching institution, often a resident or a fellow may see the patient.

Who Are Residents or Fellows?

Following medical school, a physician typically spends 3 years in residency. If the doctor decides on oncology as a specialty, the physician spends another 3 years working in oncology under the tutelage of experienced oncologists before the physician can practice independently.

Following a review of the records, the resident or fellow will conduct the patient interview, during which the patient's history and current situation are reviewed and his or her concerns are defined. A physical examination completes the first phase of the consultation.

The resident or fellow then will present the case to the attending oncologist, and the patient will finally meet the physician he or she came to see. The attending physician probably will ask more questions and perhaps conduct another physical examination. This is another chance for the patient to ask questions. If all of the information noted above has been provided, the consultant will be able to give a second opinion on the treatment options.

■ Important Points

It is evident that the consultation can be a lengthy process. Patients should allow enough time so that they do not feel rushed. Be patient!

The purpose of the interview is to understand the sequence of events surrounding the diagnosis and treatment. Questions should be answered directly. The patient's ability to provide that information will save everyone a lot of time.

If the patient relies on the opinion of someone specific, such as a friend, spouse, or family member, bring that person along so that all of the questions can be answered at once. A lot of information is discussed and sometimes a second pair of ears is useful. Consider taping the consultation so that it can be replayed either to recall things that were missed or for someone who could not be there.

■ Surgical Decisions

For many types of cancer, surgery remains the mainstay of treatment. Tumors that have discrete borders and are located in an accessible area most likely will be removed. For example, a breast or colonic mass usually can be visualized directly when the skin and muscle over the area are retracted.

On the other hand, bronchoalveolar lung cancer presents as diffuse disease throughout the lung and cannot be removed without resecting the entire lung. If the disease is confined to one lung, a pneumonectomy (removal of a lung) may be done. However, if both lungs are involved, surgery is not an option. Some surgeries, such as for gastric cancer, can be very complicated. For example, if it is necessary to remove the stomach, part of the bowel will be pulled up to serve in place of the stomach. Whatever surgery is recommended for the diagnosis, patients may want to get another opinion from a surgeon who performs many cancer surgeries. It is important to bring the actual films of the CT scans so that the surgeon can clearly see the disease that has been identified radiographically. Sometimes additional radiographic studies may be done in the operating room during the surgery. This is known as **intraoperative** testing.

Lymph nodes in the area of the primary tumor will be removed so that they can be examined for microscopic disease. The surgeon will palpate the surgical field for other possible areas of disease that may not have been identified on CT. For example, when the abdomen is opened to remove the primary tumor, the surgeon will be able to visualize and palpate the liver. Small lesions (less than 1 cm) may not been seen on CT scan but will be seen by direct visualization. If there are fewer than four lesions in the liver, the surgeon may opt to resect them during the surgery.

■ New Procedures

Surgical procedures, just like other forms of treatment, are always under study to improve processes and outcomes. Just as cholecystectomy (removal of the gallbladder) was a major operation in the past, most are now done by a laparoscopic approach. In this case, a round hollow tube (laparoscope) is introduced into the abdomen through a small incision. Because the entire surgery can be accomplished through the scope, the procedure is much less traumatic to the patient than the large incision and tissue manipulation of years past. Recovery from laparoscopic surgery is easier and faster than recovery from a major surgical procedure.

Similarly, some cancer surgeries can be performed using the same technique. Most often, laparoscopic surgery may be used in early disease where visualization and palpation of a large area is not necessary. An experienced surgeon is the best judge of whether that approach is appropriate.

Another procedure currently under investigation is cryosurgery, where a few small lesions, for example, in the liver, are frozen. Through an abdominal incision, a probe is placed directly into the tumor, and the cells are frozen and destroyed. This procedure can be used only if there are fewer than four lesions that are small in size.

Radiofrequency ablation (RFA) uses the same criteria as cryosurgery, i.e., there can only be a few small lesions. However, this procedure is actually a process in which the lesions are heated and destroyed. This procedure is done by a radiologist.

Cryosurgery or RFA will be used if the liver is the *only* site of metastatic disease. With removal of the primary tumor and the addition of one of these procedures, all known disease has been removed. If there are other sites of metastatic disease, it is not wise to expose the patient to the possible complications of the procedures if all of the disease cannot be removed.

■ Radiation Decisions

Radiation is defined as the use of gamma rays to achieve death of the cells. It can be given as **external beam radiation,** in which the beam is delivered to a specific site at levels high enough to kill tumor cells with minimal damage to surrounding tissue. This therapy typically is done daily for several weeks in an outpatient setting.

During the initial visit, called the **simulation,** the exact site to be radiated is identified and tattoos are placed on the skin to ensure the correct location is radiated each time. The total dose is determined and then **fractionated** so that a small dose is given every day, usually Monday through Friday, in order to control the side effects.

External beam radiation can cause irritation, similar to a bad sunburn, to the skin overlying the radiated area. Depending on which internal structures are within the radiation field, other side effects can occur, such as nausea, diarrhea, or low blood counts.

Radiation can be delivered internally (called **brachytherapy**) by radioactive beads or pins that are placed inside the body. During surgery, small plastic tubes are placed in the area to be radiated. Radioactive beads or pins are placed in the tubes. Patients are hospitalized during the treatment, which lasts a few days, and must be isolated to protect others from the radioactivity.

Radiation is used in many different ways in the treatment of cancer.

- Neoadjuvant: before surgery
  - Used before surgery to reduce the size of the mass and improve surgical outcome
- Adjuvant: in the absence of known disease
  - Used after the primary tumor has been removed to treat possible remaining tumor cells or unknown micrometastases
- Curative: given with the intent to effect a cure
  - Used in certain cancers, such as prostate cancer, as primary treatment
- Palliative: given when all disease cannot be removed
  - Used to treat one specific site of metastasis when there are other known sites
  - Used to treat painful bony metastasis
  - Used to treat soft tissue lesions involving a nerve or spinal cord and causing pain or loss of motor ability

Neoadjuvant Therapy

In certain cancers, such as esophageal or rectal cancer, radiation sometimes is used to reduce the size of the tumor before surgery. In the case of a large mass, some believe that using radiation first will shrink the size of the tumor and, therefore, may allow a better surgical outcome.

Sometimes chemotherapy is given concurrently with radiation as a **radiosensitizer.** Certain chemotherapy drugs make cells more sensitive to radiation.

Adjuvant Therapy

When all of the known cancer has been surgically resected, adjuvant radiation sometimes is recommended. In some early-stage diseases, such as stage I breast cancer, previous clinical testing has shown that surgery plus radiation is adequate treatment. In other cases, the decision is based either on the natural history of some cancers, such as rectal cancer, or on other factors that increase the chance of recurrence. In some situations, patients may receive both neoadjuvant radiation before surgery and then adjuvant radiation after surgical resection.

Use of radiation is limited by dose and location. As discussed earlier, some areas of the body cannot be radiated without causing damage to vital structures that underlie the target location. For example, to radiate the pancreas, the beam would have to pass through the bowel. Achieving a high enough dose of radiation to treat the pancreas would cause permanent and irreversible damage to the bowel, and the damage could be life-threatening. Similarly, the amount of radiation that can be delivered to an area is limited for the same reason. Radiating above that limit can cause more damage than good.

At the completion of radiation therapy, a report, called the *radiation summary,* is generated. This report describes in detail the site, dose, and duration of the treatment. It is important to obtain a copy of the radiation summary and retain it in the patient's personal file. If, at some later time, the doctor is considering radiation as a treatment option, the summary will help to clarify if that is a possibility.

■ Chemotherapy Decisions

The word **chemotherapy** carries with it many negative connotations. But, strictly speaking, taking two aspirins for a headache is chemotherapy. Any time a drug is used to treat a symptom or condition, that is chemotherapy. However, the common use of the term represents the drugs that are used to treat cancers. This class of drugs often is referred to as *cytotoxic,* meaning they are toxic to cells.

Chemotherapy can be used in many ways in the treatment of various cancers. Depending on the type of cancer and its stage, chemotherapy can cure, keep the cancer from spreading, slow the growth, or relieve symptoms.

Single Agent versus Combination Therapy

When used alone as a single agent, few drugs demonstrate significant results against cancer. Most often, drugs are used in combination therapies. How to combine drugs to create effective regimens is often the objective of clinical trials. Typically, drugs with different mechanisms of action and side-effect profiles are combined. In that way, the cancer cells are attacked in different ways without causing unacceptable toxicity. For example, Drug A may interrupt cell division by interfering with chromosome division, while Drug B may interfere with helix formation after chromosome replication has taken place. In this way, cell division is potentially altered by two different mechanisms, leading to greater efficacy than either drug used independently.

Understanding the side-effect profile of each drug in a combination is important. For example, Drug A may cause diarrhea as the most significant toxicity, while Drug B's toxicity is myelosuppression, lowering of the blood counts.

Some drugs are used in combination with other drugs that potentiate them. For example, calcium leucovorin is a mineral that, when given with 5-fluorouracil (5-FU), can increase the efficacy of 5-FU. Leucovorin is not a cytotoxic drug; rather, in this case, it is a **sensitizer.**

Leucovorin also is used, in some cases, as a chemo **protectant.** Methotrexate, when given in high doses, can cause severe toxicity. However, using leucovorin following the administration of methotrexate (leucovorin rescue) avoids this reaction. Other drugs that are not cytotoxic also function as chemo sensitizers or chemo protectants. Similarly, cytotoxic drugs can serve as sensitizers. Recall the discussion on the use of chemotherapy as a radiation sensitizer.

Dose and Frequency of Treatment

The dose used in treatment is determined in phase I clinical trials (see Chapter 5 for an in-depth discussion). The prevailing theory is to deliver the highest dose possible without causing unacceptable side effects. This theory, based on the assumption that more is better, may not always be true.

Similarly, the frequency with which a drug is given also is determined in a phase I trial. The objectives of chemotherapy schedules are to

- Maintain adequate drug levels to control tumor growth
- Avoid unacceptable toxicities

Therefore, some single agent regimens will provide for a drug to be given daily for 5 consecutive days and then no treatment for the next 3 weeks. Other regimens will dictate that the drug be given weekly, every 3 weeks, or every 6 weeks. In some cases, the drug is given weekly for 4 consecutive weeks, followed by a 2-week rest.

In combination regimens, different drugs may be given on different days to maximize efficacy and minimize toxicity. Table 3-1 gives an example of such a regimen.

Table 3-1	Example of Treatment Regimen
Drug	**Frequency**
Drug A	Day 1, 8, 5, 22
Drug B	Day 1, 8
Drug C	Day 1, 22

Methods of Delivery

Chemotherapy can be delivered to the patient through a variety of routes. Most often, treatment is given **systemically,** meaning that it will go throughout the body. This is accomplished via an oral route (by mouth) or an intravenous route (i.v.), which is through a needle in the vein.

Intravenous delivery of drugs can be given through a peripheral line or a central line. A peripheral i.v. is placed in a superficial vein in the patient's hand or arm and is removed after each treatment.

Percutaneous intravenous central catheter (PICC) lines are long catheters that are placed in the arm by specially trained nurses. PICCs require daily attention to change dressings and keep the line patent. Because the catheter exits through an opening in the skin, great care must be exercised to avoid infection. These catheters generally are used for short-term therapy (1 to 2 months) and removed.

Central lines **(Port-a-Cath)** are placed during an outpatient surgical procedure and remain in place for extended periods of time Fig. 3-1).

Port-a-Caths are usually placed under the skin with the diaphragm secured to the chest wall. In some cases, the central line is placed in the arm. Either way, the catheter is threaded into a large vein. Because the skin is closed over the diaphragm, the chance of infection is less than with a PICC. The Port-a-Cath is accessed using a special right-angle needle under sterile technique.

Groshong Catheter

Another type of **central venous catheter** placed as an outpatient procedure is the Groshong catheter. The catheter has two lines that remain outside of the patient's body. These lines, which are narrow tubes with rubber caps on the end, are threaded through the chest wall into the largest vein in the body (the superior vena cava). Blood can be drawn out of either tube, and medications and blood products can be given through the tubes. Because there are two tubes, patients with Groshong catheters can receive two different medications at the

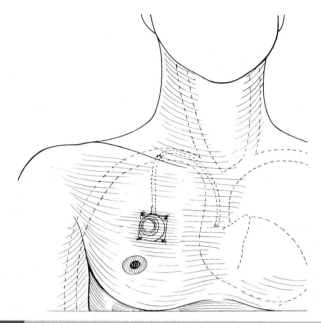

Figure 3-1 Port-a-Cath

same time. Groshong catheters are typically the catheter of choice for patients with leukemia.

Catheters afford the patient the ability to receive frequent treatment without multiple needle sticks and damage to the veins. Blood can be drawn from these lines for blood tests, even after treatment is complete. Because the catheter has direct communication to the patient's circulatory system, there is a greater danger of infection than with a simple peripheral blood draw. Therefore, catheters are entered under sterile technique and, by law, require nurses rather than laboratory technicians to access them.

Certain chemotherapy drugs have the potential to cause serious damage to the skin if the drug leaks from the vein (*extravasates* or *infiltrates*) into the surrounding tissue. Some cancer centers require that patients receiving drugs with this potential *(vesicants)* must have a central line.

Central-line catheters have helped to reduce some of the trauma associated with chemotherapy treatments. There are possible complications associated with the placement and maintenance of these catheters. Discuss the advantages and disadvantages of a central-line catheter with the physician, treatment nurse, and other patients before deciding whether or not to get one.

Intraperitoneal Catheter

In some diseases that are contained within the abdomen, one treatment option is to instill chemotherapy directly into the abdominal cavity **(intraperitoneal therapy),** in essence, to wash the surface of the pelvic cavity (peritoneum) with chemotherapy. The catheter(s) is placed during surgery and remains in place for the duration of the therapy, usually a week or two.

Omaya Reservoir

In some diseases, the cerebrospinal fluid (the fluid that surrounds the spinal column and brain) is found to contain malignant cells. Instillation of chemotherapy into the spinal column **(intrathecal therapy),** is an important treatment option. This therapy can be delivered via a needle placed into the back between the vertebrae. However, after several treatments, scar tissue can form, which makes placement of the needle through the back difficult or impossible. For patients requiring frequent therapy into the spinal canal, an Omaya reservoir is placed in the patient's head. Similar to a Port-a-Cath, the diaphragm is placed under the scalp and the catheter is threaded into the spinal canal.

■ Types of Chemotherapy

Adjuvant Therapy

When all of the known cancer is surgically resected, chemotherapy may be given as an adjuvant treatment. Recall from the section on radiation that adjuvant therapy is given to treat any possible micrometastases. In some cancers, it is known that the use of adjuvant chemotherapy reduces the likelihood of the cancer returning at a later time.

Therapy to Control Disease

When all of the known cancer cells cannot be surgically removed (unresectable), chemotherapy is given to treat the existing disease. The ability of chemotherapy to cure metastatic disease has not been proven. Rather, cytotoxic drugs traditionally are used to keep the known disease from growing and spreading.

Palliative Therapy

When unresectable, metastatic disease is diffuse, chemotherapy sometimes is used to control symptoms such as pain. If the disease is very advanced, the benefits of chemotherapy versus the side effects experienced by the patient must be weighed carefully to determine what is in the best interest of the patient.

Duration of Therapy

Before treatment is initiated, the patient's cancer is staged to establish the extent of the disease. This is done using CT scans, bone scans, or, in some cases, tumor markers. After a specified number of treatments, the patient's cancer is restaged using exactly the same testing procedures so that the extent of the disease can be compared to the earlier study. If the disease is stable, meaning no growth, or, better yet, if the disease has responded to the treatment by becoming smaller, then the therapy is believed to be working and treatment with the same drugs will continue. If, however, the disease has grown, the current treatment is determined not to be working and a change in therapy is recommended.

Response to therapy is unpredictable. Individuals with the same diagnoses often do not respond equally to a drug. One person could have a complete response, meaning all known disease has disappeared, while the next person could have no response at all. However, the second person could, in turn, respond to the next drug(s) used.

Sometimes treatment is stopped because of side effects (toxicities) caused by the drugs. Most often, holding treatment for a week or two or reducing the dose of the chemotherapy is enough to allow the side effects to abate. However, sometimes the side effects can be severe, such as diarrhea that leads to dehydration or lowering of blood counts that take weeks to recover. When the side effects outweigh the benefits of the treatment, the physician generally will decide to try another treatment.

As long as the disease continues to respond to therapy and the side effects caused by the drugs are tolerated, the same treatment regimen is continued.

■ Treatment Decision Continuum

Decisions regarding treatment are not a one-time experience for a cancer patient. As described earlier, if and when one treatment no longer is effective, new options are presented and another decision about treatment must be made. Every patient is faced with the same options:

- Wait and watch
- Standard therapy

- Experimental therapy
- Alternative therapy
- Supportive care

Wait and Watch

What does wait and watch mean? Does it mean that the doctor feels that treatment is futile? Certainly not!

Adjuvant therapy (treatment given when all known disease has been resected) typically is given for a specified period of time. At the end of the prescribed therapy, the patient's cancer is restaged and, if no disease is found, watchful waiting usually is recommended. This means the patient undergoes blood tests and doctor visits at certain intervals that are determined by the length of time since treatment ended.

Although one would think that the end of therapy with no evidence of disease should be great news for a patient, there are times when the patient may feel "separation anxiety." For some patients, knowing that the medical team is examining them and checking blood counts on a regular basis is reassuring. Every symptom, no matter how insignificant, is addressed during regular visits. Now, the next visit may be 3 months away and what if . . . .

Remember that the medical team is only a phone call away. They understand the patient's fear and are willing to talk on the phone or see the patient if a symptom arises.

The other side of the coin is the patient who is only too happy to see the end of therapy and wants to forget that this nasty episode ever happened. That patient may ignore follow-up recommendations. Most patients are somewhere in between.

Watchful waiting is a recommendation in another scenario. For example, a patient with a small amount of known disease has been receiving chemotherapy for several months. Each set of scans has shown that the disease has not been growing. However, the patient's blood counts have been consistently low, requiring dose reductions and frequently skipped treatments. In this case, the physician may recommend stopping therapy, watching the disease to be sure that the tumors do not begin to grow, and waiting for the bone marrow to recover.

In some patients, the natural history of the disease may show periods of slow growth or no growth at all. Weighing the benefits of therapy against the side effects is always a consideration. Depending on the circumstances, these patients would be followed more closely than patients with no known disease.

Standard Therapy

In many diseases, there is a specified treatment regimen that is recommended as first-line therapy. For some diseases, if the first therapy is not successful, there are additional drugs, called *second-line therapy,* that are generally recommended. These treatment regimens, utilizing United States **Food and Drug Administration (FDA)-** approved drugs either as single agents or in combination, are called *standard therapy.* New regimens are defined by clinical trials that compare the current standard therapy to new therapies. When making treatment decisions, a patient may be presented with more than one option and will feel confused about which therapy is "best." What is truly best is what works, and that varies from patient to patient. The final decision about treatment rests with the patient. Comparing treatment schedules and side-effect profiles may help a patient to choose.

For standard therapy regimens, the physician is able to quote response rates and discuss side-effect profiles. The response rate is given as a percentage. For example, if the regimen has a 20% response rate, that means 20 of every 100 patients who receive this regimen will have some response to the treatment. The response may be complete disappearance of all tumors, reduction in the size of some or all of the tumors, decrease in tumor marker values, and/or improvement in the quality of life. Sometimes, the benefit of treatment may be measured in time to progression (how long before the disease grows after starting therapy) or in time to survival (how long the average patient survives after diagnosis).

In some diseases, there is no known therapy that has proved to be effective. In such cases, some physicians will recommend treatment with FDA-approved drugs, while others will suggest that patients in this situation seek experimental therapy. Sometimes, the patient may be told that because there is no effective treatment known for his or her disease, no treatment is recommended. At that point, the patient's value system (as discussed earlier) must dictate the next step.

Experimental Therapy

Experimental therapy can be divided into two categories:

1. New combinations of known treatment modalities or drugs
2. Investigational treatments or drugs

New Combinations of Approved Drugs

A few drugs are effective when given as a single agent, but often efficacy can be increased or enhanced when drugs are combined.

Typically, two or more drugs are given together; this is known as *combination therapy*. The decision to combine drugs is determined by several factors:

- The drugs may work by different mechanisms.
- The drugs have different toxicities.
- One drug improves the efficacy of the other.
- One drug ameliorates the side effects of the other.
- The response rate and/or time to progression is improved.
- The survival time is prolonged.

Understanding cell metabolism would require an in-depth lesson in cell biology. In simple terms, in order for cells to replicate, they undergo a process during which the genes synthesize or duplicate themselves. Drugs work by interrupting that process at a variety of points. Over time, cancer cells can mutate to compensate for the interruption caused by a drug and essentially outsmart the drug. Combining cytotoxic drugs (drugs that kill tumor cells) that work by different mechanisms keeps cancer cells off balance and may delay or thwart the mutation process. It also is believed that attacking cancer cells by more than one approach may prove to be more effective than single agent therapy. When designing combination therapy, the side effects of the cytotoxic drugs must be considered to avoid overlapping toxicities. For example, if two drugs both cause diarrhea as the primary side effect, combining them could cause intolerable toxicity. Sometimes, modifying doses when combining drugs will help control side effects. The toxicity profile is analyzed carefully when new combinations are being tested.

Another reason to combine drugs is to create a synergistic effect. Occasionally, a drug that has very little efficacy as a single agent will potentiate another drug. Oxaliplatin, an experimental cytotoxic drug used in the treatment of metastatic colorectal cancer, has only 10% efficacy as a single agent (1). However, when it is combined with 5-FU, the combination has approximately 20% efficacy in patients who have already progressed through 5-FU therapy (2). Sometimes, synergy can be effected through the use of a noncytotoxic drug combined with a cytotoxic drug. Calcium leucovorin, a mineral, when combined with 5-FU for the treatment of colorectal cancer, increases the number of patients who respond versus patients given 5-FU as a single agent (3).

At other times, combining drugs will allow higher, and presumably more effective, doses of a drug to be given. Leucovorin is used as a "rescue" treatment for methotrexate. When given in high doses, methotrexate causes severe toxicity, making it intolerable. However, when methotrexate is followed by leucovorin, the side effects are ameliorated.

Investigational Drugs

Finding or developing new drugs to improve and prolong lives is the focus of scientists and pharmaceutical companies worldwide. Sometimes drugs are made from natural resources, such as paclitaxel (Taxol), which originally was developed from the bark of the Chinese yew tree. Because of the scarcity of these trees and, therefore, the drug, scientists finally learned how to synthesize the drug. Researchers continue to work with new molecules to develop new drugs.

Sometimes, drugs developed years ago but shelved because of toxicities are being retrieved from closets of research laboratories and revisited. The drug Camptosar (irinotecan hydrochloride), used in the treatment of colorectal cancer, has such a history. The parent compound originally was developed from a tree known as *Camptotheca acuminata*. The original drug, camptothecin, was tested in the 1960s but caused severe toxicity and was abandoned. In the 1980s, researchers took another look at the drug. By attaching another molecular chain, the compound became a semisynthetic drug that is more soluble and, therefore, more tolerable than the earlier compound. Interestingly, when molecular chains were attached to the parent compound at different locations, the resulting molecules created two additional compounds, topotecan and 9-aminocamptothecin, which are active in the treatment of various cancers (4).

Alternative Therapy

For some people, the poor cure rate associated with solid tumor treatments is not acceptable. Believing traditional treatment causes devastating side effects with little hope for complete success, people look for alternative methods of treatment. Sometimes, treatment consists of supplemental herbs, minerals, and vitamins. Other times, treatment includes intravenous infusions of untested compounds, coffee enemas, and various other methods.

Because many of our approved drugs are plant derivatives, taking plant extracts typically is not harmful and may, in fact, have some benefit. If a patient is taking nutritional supplements in addition to standard therapy, it is important to discuss these supplements with the treating physician to be sure that the supplements do not interfere with treatment. For example, 5-FU is a folate antagonist, meaning it interferes with the cell's metabolism of folic acid. Patients should not take vitamin B_1, folic acid, while taking 5-FU.

Many alternative therapies tout their success through testimonials from patients who were "cured." It is important to look at such information. Researchers know that the natural history of some cancers includes periods of slow growth or no growth at all. Physicians agree that if a treatment has been successful in one or several patients, then it should be subjected to the rigors of clinical trials to prove its efficacy.

Great care must be taken to avoid unscrupulous people who appeal to patients' hopes and fears. Often alternative therapies cost patients not only a great deal of money, but also precious time that could be spent receiving treatments with known efficacy.

> **Note:**
>
> For more information on questionable cancer therapies, visit *http://www.quackwatch.com*. The American Cancer Society (ACS) also can supply position papers on questionable therapies. Patients can call their local ACS office or 1-800-227-2345. Advice also is available from the Candlelighters Childhood Cancer Foundation Ombudsman's program at 1-301-657-8401 and the National Council Against Health Fraud at 1-909-824-4690 (5).

■ References

1. Becouarn Y, Ychou M, Ducreux M, et al., for the French Federation Nationale des Centres de Lutte Contre le Cancer. Oxaliplatin (L-OHP) as first-line chemotherapy in metastatic colorectal cancer (MCRC) patients: preliminary activity/toxicity report. *Proc Am Soc Clin Oncol* 1997;16:abst 803,228a.
2. Gerard B, Bleiberg H, Michel J, et al. Oxaliplatin combined to 5-FU and folinic acid (5FU/FA) as second- or third-line treatment in patients with advanced colorectal cancer (CRC). *Proc Am Soc Clin Oncol* 1997;16:abst 1025,288a.
3. Leichman CG, Fleming TR, Muggia FM, et al. Phase II study of fluorouracil and its modulation in advanced colorectal cancer: a Southwest Oncology Group study. *J Clin Oncol* 1995;13:1303–1311.
4. Wall ME, Wani MC. Camptothecin: discovery to clinic. *Ann N Y Acad Sci* 1998;802:1–12.
5. Barrett S, Herbert V. Questionable cancer therapies. Available at *http://www.quackwatch.com/01QuackeryRelatedTopics/cancer.html*. Accessed August 10, 2000.

CHAPTER 4

Drug Development

Drug development is a lengthy and costly process, similar to looking for the famous needle in the haystack. Every year, 5,000 compounds enter preclinical testing, but only five of those drugs make it to human testing. A compound may not show any efficacy or may have such devastating toxicities that it is not safe for human use. Researchers will attempt to chemically and structurally modify the drug to overcome the limitations, but if that is not possible, the drug may be abandoned.

Of the five drugs that are tested in humans, only one of those drugs actually is approved by the United States Food and Drug Administration (FDA) for commercial use. The entire process from preclinical testing to FDA approval takes from 8 to 12 years to complete. According to a 1993 report by the Congressional Office of Technology Assessment, the average cost of developing a drug is $359 million (1,2).

The process of identifying one new drug requires the expertise of many different disciplines. In the past, organic chemists, physiologists, and statisticians made up the research team. In recent years, the team has been expanded to include new members:

- Biochemists, who study the chemistry of life processes
- Molecular biologists, who study the molecules that make up living matter

- Toxicologists, who investigate compounds' potential for harm in animal models
- Pharmacologists, who look at how the drugs work
- Computer scientists, who use their sophisticated machines to analyze and assess new chemicals (3)

■ Sources of New Compounds

New medicines are either derived from natural sources, such as plants, or created in the laboratory *(synthetic compounds)*. Some drugs are a combination of natural sources that are modified in the laboratory, making them *semisynthetic*. The number of compounds that can be produced from basically the same chemical structure can number into the hundreds of millions (2).

■ New Drug Developers

Drug development is done in a variety of places. All major academic medical centers have physicians who are dedicated to laboratory development and testing of new molecules and compounds that have potential for human use. There are innumerable biotechnology companies that also are working to develop new, useful drugs. Many pharmaceutical companies have oncology divisions that spend a large amount of their resources on research and development of new drugs. Often, the early development of drugs is begun at the biotechnology company level. Then, as a drug begins to show promise, either the compound or the entire company is purchased by a larger pharmaceutical company for further development. These decisions are economically based, because small biotechnology companies have limited sources of revenue and the costs of clinical trials are prohibitive. With the financial support of a company that has other successful drugs providing income, the costs of continued testing and development of a promising drug become more manageable.

■ Process of New Drug Development

The goal is to identify new molecules with the potential to produce a desired change in a biologic system. Some of the desired characteristics are to

- Inhibit or stimulate an important enzyme
- Alter a metabolic pathway
- Change cellular structure (2)

All drug testing begins in the laboratory, i.e., preclinical testing. **Preclinical studies** provide the initial information on the efficacy and safety of the new compound. The compound undergoes several kinds of testing, including

- Biologic screening and pharmacologic testing
- Pharmaceutical dosage formulation and stability testing
- Toxicology and safety testing

Preclinical testing can take from 3.5 to 6.5 years to complete (1,4).

Understanding the Pharmacology of a Compound

In order to explore the pharmacologic activity and therapeutic potential of a new compound, it is tested in a variety of mediums, such as tumor cell lines that are created from human malignancies and tumors that are implanted in mice. Testing done on laboratory models is called *in vitro* and testing done in living organisms is known as *in vivo.* Computer models also are used to glean information about the compound.

As a drug is broken down in the body, the resulting chemical components are called **metabolites.** Sometimes the metabolite is more potent than the parent compound and, in fact, may be the active ingredient. Understanding what the metabolites are, how they work, and how long it takes to excrete them from the body is an important part of the pharmacologic studies.

As the testing proceeds, modifications are made to the original compound to improve pharmacologic activity. The goal is to find the compound with the most therapeutic promise and the least potentially harmful properties.

Formulation and Dosing

The next step in the process is to put the compound into a form and strength that is suitable for human consumption. A drug can be developed in one or more dosage forms, such as liquid, tablets, capsules, ointments, sprays, and patches. The strength of the drug typically is determined in milligrams (i.e., 5, 10, 20, 50, or 500). In the final formulation, the drug is combined with other ingredients known as **excipients.** Excipients may be necessary to provide stability to the compound, affect absorption, improve the taste of an oral drug, or be used in any other number of circumstances to improve the ability of the drug to be used in humans. Excipients also must be tested for any potential reactions in humans. Sometimes, patients may be allergic or have a side effect caused by the excipient and not the drug.

Toxicity and Safety

Drugs that show some activity in mice tumor models go on for toxicity testing in at least two animal species. Toxicity and safety testing is done to determine the potential risk of the compound to both humans and the environment. At this point, the compound is tested again in animals and other test systems to determine the relationship among the dose, the frequency of administration, and the duration of exposure. After an effective dose is found, the scientists continue to escalate the dose to identify the toxicity profile of the drug. It is expected that the toxicities noted in the animals may be anticipated in humans. However, the toxicity and dosing schedules in humans will not be fully understood until the drug is tested in phase I clinical trials.

Dose escalation in the animal studies also identifies the *lethal dose* of the drug, that is, the amount of drug that causes death of the animals. This information is used to identify the starting dose for human trials.

Consider the hypothetical situation of the experimental drug MM112. Over the course of the animal study, the mice were given the drug at escalating doses until the implanted tumors disappeared. Dosing began at 10 mg per kilogram of body weight, and the response was seen at 100 mg per kilogram. This was called the *effective dose* in mice. Dose escalation then continued to determine the dose at which the drug became lethal, i.e., the dose at which 10% of the mice died. The human starting dose typically is calculated to be 10% of the dose that killed 10% of the mice. Clearly, the starting dose for human trials is likely to be *subtherapeutic,* meaning that it is not expected to elicit a positive response in human tumors. Trials are started at low doses in case unexpected toxicities are seen. Patient safety is the foremost concern.

An important piece of information is the cause of death in the sacrificed mice. For example, if the drug causes a decrease in white blood cells and blood in the urine in animals, these same toxicities may be seen in humans. The lethal toxicity in the mice may have been renal failure (the kidneys stopped producing urine) caused by hemorrhage in the kidneys. In human testing, patients will be monitored very closely for renal toxicities. However, it is possible that the toxicities seen in humans may not relate at all to those seen in animal studies.

■ Investigational New Drug Application

Once a potentially effective compound has been identified and completed testing, the company files an application to the FDA for an **Investigational New Drug (IND)** number. The purpose of the application is to give the FDA all known information about the drug supporting the premise that it is reasonable to begin human testing (5). It also describes the company's plan for the clinical (human) research, including the specific **protocol** for a phase I study.

Once the FDA approves the application, an IND number is issued and human testing can begin. Simultaneously, the company contracts a manufacturer to produce sufficient quantities of the drug to begin human testing. When the FDA receives an IND application, the agency requests an inspection of the manufacturing facilities. Nearly 15,000 establishments in the United States manufacture, test, pack, and label drug products for human consumption. The Federal Food, Drug, and Cosmetic Act requires the FDA to inspect these facilities at least once every 2 years. The investigators must determine that the data in the application are authentic and accurate and that good manufacturing practices are being used (6).

> **Important Note:**
>
> Researchers have been very successful in curing cancer in mice. Unfortunately, these successes often have not translated to humans. It is a huge leap of faith to believe that a drug that shows impressive results in the laboratory will show similar results in cancer patients. Responsible researchers will emphasize that information to patients anticipating participation in phase I and phase II clinical trials.

■ References

1. Washington Biotechnology & Medical Technology Online. Drug development & approval process. Available at *http://www.wabio.com/dis/drug_approv .htm*. Accessed November 29, 2000.
2. The drug development and approval process. Available at *http://www .mhsource.com/resource/process.html*. Accessed November 29, 2000.
3. FDA consumer special report. The beginnings: laboratory and animal studies. Available at *http://www.fda.gov/fdac/special/newdrug/begin.html*. Accessed November 29, 2000.

4. Alliance Pharmaceutical Corp. Phases of product development. Available at *http://www.allp.con/drug_dev.htm*. Accessed November 29, 2000.

5. Center for Drug Evaluation and Research. Drug applications. Available at *http://www.fda.gov/cder/about/smallbiz/faq.htm*. Accessed November 29, 2000.

6. FDA consumer special report. An inside look at FDA on-site. Available at *http://www.fda.gov/fdac/special/newdrug/onsite.html*. Accessed November 29, 2000.

CHAPTER 5

Clinical Trials

When a compound shows potential in preclinical testing, the company that developed the drug will proceed with human testing, known as a **clinical trial.** Step one is writing the protocol. A protocol is a written statement of the rationale, objectives, and procedures to conduct a clinical trial. Typically, the protocol is written with oversight of the medical monitor, the physician at the company who is responsible for all matters related to that particular drug. In the language of the protocol, the company becomes known as the **sponsor.** Once completed, the protocol is sent to one or more cancer centers that will execute the protocol. The physician at the cancer center who is in charge of the study is called the **principal investigator** (PI). Other physicians who help to identify and treat study patients are called co-investigators. The person who handles all of the details of the study (in oncology, this is typically a nurse) is called the **study coordinator** or **clinical research coordinator.** Depending on the size of the cancer center and the number of studies done there, additional personnel at the cancer center may be involved, such as a **data manager,** who assists the study coordinator and records the data. Overall, the execution of a protocol involves many people at many different levels to ensure that the patients are safe and the study is properly run. This will be discussed more in later chapters.

Every protocol is organized in a similar fashion:

- Background
- Objectives
- Study design
- Inclusion and exclusion criteria
- Study procedures
- Adverse events

■ Background

The background begins with a statement of the problem. For example, if the protocol is looking at a drug for lung cancer, this section will discuss the prevalence, incidence, and survival statistics associated with the disease. Current treatments will be reviewed, with a statement that there is need for improvement in response or survival rates.

The drug is introduced with details about its chemical structure and preclinical antitumor activity. Information about all aspects of the animal testing is discussed in detail, together with all of the safety data. All of this information supports the rationale for this particular study.

■ Objectives

The hypothesis is established, and the primary and secondary objectives outline exactly what the protocol is designed to determine. For example, in a phase I, dose-finding study, the primary objective might be stated as follows:

> Define the maximum tolerated dose of Drug A when given weekly via intravenous administration.

Secondary objectives for the above study might include determining tumor response to Drug A and defining the **pharmacokinetics** (how Drug A is metabolized).

■ Study Design

The protocol design must scientifically prove the objectives while also providing for patient safety. For example, in a phase I study, in which a drug is tested for the first time in humans, the study design might state that three patients will be treated at each dose level, with an increase in dose only after all three patients have taken the drug for 4 weeks and no serious side effects are seen. It might further state that each patient must complete 1 week of taking the drug before the next patient can be treated. In that way, any unexpected toxicity (side effect) will expose the minimum number of people at any one time.

The study design also will define the number of patients to be treated during the study. In a phase II or phase III clinical trial, the statistician specifies the number of subjects needed to prove the hypothesis and make the data statistically significant. In a phase I study, it is impossible to predetermine exactly how many subjects will be treated before the maximum tolerated dose is defined. Therefore, most phase I studies are written to have 30 participants, but the number can be increased or decreased if necessary.

■ Inclusion and Exclusion Criteria

The **inclusion/exclusion criteria** define the patient selection parameters for participation in the study. Table 5-1 shows a sample of an inclusion/exclusion page of a phase II protocol.

In summary, the patients must be adults with colorectal cancer that has spread outside the colon and who have not received treatment for the metastatic disease. A tissue biopsy must prove that the patient's cancer is adenocarcinoma. The disease must be able to be reliably measured by serial evaluations either by computerized tomography (CT) scan or x-ray film or by a reliable tumor marker (such as prostate-specific antigen [PSA] in the case of prostate cancer), or be palpable so that it can be measured during a physical examination. For example, a patient who had all of the disease surgically removed would not be eligible for the study. In this study, the objective is to determine if the drug will effectively treat colorectal cancer. If there is no disease to follow, there is no way to measure efficacy.

Because no one knows what effect the study drug might have on unborn fetuses, patients who have childbearing potential must agree to practice responsible birth control. A baseline pregnancy test must be performed in all female patients who have not been surgically sterilized or who are not several years beyond their last menstrual period.

Patients must comply with the study requirements, that is, have blood tests as ordered, take treatment on schedule, and keep appointments. Patients who comply with all study requirements are known as **evaluable patients.** It is important that a patient understands this responsibility prior to agreeing to participate in the study. Failure to do so results in nonevaluable patients and can compromise the results of the study.

Table 5-1	Inclusion/Exclusion Criteria

Inclusion Criteria

The answer must be YES to the following statements for a patient to be eligible.

1. The patient is at least 18 years of age.
2. The patient has untreated metastatic colorectal cancer. The patient may have had adjuvant therapy, but no treatment for metastatic disease.
3. The patient must have histologically proven adenocarcinoma.
4. The patient must have measurable or evaluable disease (radiographic measurement, serum tumor marker, or physical clinical measurement). Patients without evidence of disease are excluded from the study.
5. Male or female. Female patients must agree to use effective contraception, be surgically sterile, or be postmenopausal. Male patients must agree to use barrier contraception or be surgically sterile. All at-risk female patients must have a negative serum pregnancy test within 7 days prior to study drug administration.
6. Patient must be willing and able to comply with all study requirements. The patient or a legally authorized representative must fully understand all elements of the informed consent and have signed the informed consent.

Exclusion Criteria

The answer must be NO to the following statements for the patient to be eligible for the study.

1. Patient has an **absolute neutrophil count** <1,500/mm³; platelet count <100,000/mm³; hemoglobin <9.0 g/dL.
2. Patient has significant liver function abnormality as manifested by an increase in serum transaminases (AST), aspartate aminotransferase (ALT), alanine aminotransferase (ALT >3.0 × upper limit of normal or a total bilirubin >2.0 mg/dL.
3. Patient has significant renal function abnormality (serum creatinine >2 mg/dL).
4. Patient has received prior treatment for metastatic colorectal cancer.
5. Patient has a Karnofsky performance status (KPS) <70%.
6. Patient has a history of another malignancy, other than *in situ* carcinoma of the cervix or basal cell carcinoma of the skin, within the 5 years prior to study drug treatment.
7. Patient has a known intolerance to any of the excipients in the study drug formulation.
8. Patient has any other acute or chronic medical or psychiatric condition or laboratory abnormality that may increase the risks associated with study participation/study drug administration or may interfere with interpretation of the study results.

Laboratory parameters are necessary because patients with abnormal laboratory values may be at added risk when taking a study drug. If a drug is metabolized in the liver, a patient with compromised liver function could become seriously toxic. If the drug is excreted in the kidneys, lack of adequate kidney function could lead to toxicity. Similarly, a patient's **performance status** helps define the patient's ability to tolerate the treatment and the rigors of a clinical trial. Performance status percentages are defined by the patient's ability to perform certain usual tasks of daily living, such as preparing meals and personal hygiene.

Patients diagnosed with a cancer other than the one being treated by the study drug must be excluded. As an example, take the case of Mrs. Clark, who was diagnosed with breast cancer in 1997. It was surgically resected and did not need further treatment. Then, in 2000, she was diagnosed with colorectal cancer that had metastasized to her liver. From a study perspective, it may be very difficult to be sure that the liver metastases are truly from the colorectal cancer and not from the breast cancer. If this patient does not respond to the treatment, the question would be did the drug not work or was the origin of the liver metastases really from the breast cancer and not the colorectal cancer. For this reason, exclusion of patients with recent prior cancers is necessary.

In addition to each item in the inclusion and exclusion criteria, there are many other situations that might render a patient ineligible to participate in a clinical trial. Although every laboratory value is not defined, a low potassium level or a high calcium level would need to be treated before a patient could begin an experimental treatment. In many cases, once a patient has been treated successfully for the abnormality, he or she may enroll in the study.

Read the following case study and determine if the patient is eligible for the study as defined in the inclusion/exclusion criteria in Table 5-1.

■ Case Study

Jack Johnson was diagnosed with colon cancer in September 1997. At the time of his original surgery, the primary lesion in his colon and five local lymph nodes were removed. The pathology report indicated that the primary tumor and three of the five lymph nodes were positive for adenocarcinoma. No other sites of disease were found by CT scan or by the surgeon; therefore, Jack's final diagnosis was stage III colon cancer. Jack received 6 months of adjuvant chemotherapy and remained disease-free until November 1998. A rise of his tumor marker (carcinoembryonic antigen [CEA]) level concerned his oncologist and a CT scan was ordered. Unfortunately, the scan showed several small lesions in his liver.

The study is designed for patients with untreated metastatic colon cancer. Does Jack meet that criteria? Yes, he does. Originally, all of Jack's known disease was surgically removed and he received adjuvant therapy. His disease was not metastatic at that time. However, when his cancer returned in his liver, he was now considered to have metastatic disease. Jack has never been treated for metastatic disease, so he is eligible for the study.

Washout

In studies that are designed for patients who have already received other chemotherapy regimens, patients typically must wait 4 weeks after completion of the last drug before starting the experimental drug. The **washout period** is needed because nothing is known about the potential interactions between the first drug and the new drug. It is important to ensure that all of the earlier drug is out of the patient's system before introducing an experimental drug. Possible drug–drug interactions could cause serious side effects.

■ Study Procedures

The study procedures section of a protocol reads like a "to do" list. Typically, there is a whole battery of tests that must be done at various intervals during the study. The initial testing is referred to as **screening** or **baseline** and establishes the patient's eligibility for the study. After the patient is accepted into the study and treatment with the study drug begins, specific blood tests, radiographic tests, as well as vital signs (blood pressure, heart rate, respiratory rate, and temperature) and physical examinations are done at prescribed intervals. The determination of exactly which tests are done at what time is driven by concerns for patient safety. For example, if a drug demonstrated myelosuppression (lowering of the blood counts) in the earlier studies, weekly blood tests would be checked. In anticipation of such a situation, the protocol will outline steps to be taken depending on how low the counts are. For example, a small decrease in blood counts might result in reducing the dose of the study drug. The procedures section addresses all foreseeable possibilities so that all patients will be treated in exactly the same way.

Deviations from the procedures are called **protocol violations.** The sponsor and the United States Food and Drug Administration (FDA) find protocol violations unacceptable. Treating a patient who is not really eligible for the study is a serious infraction. In other cases, for example, not taking a patient's temperature is considered a minor violation. If minor infractions became common occurrences, then they are cause for concern. From a patient's perspective, not having blood tests as scheduled or not keeping scheduled appointments is a protocol violation. Patients who cause several protocol violations may be removed from a study for noncompliance. When a protocol violation occurs, the physician or study coordinator who is executing the protocol must write an acknowledgment of the violation as well as the action taken to avoid this problem in the future.

The protocol procedures dictate how to collect data to meet the objectives of the study. For example, in a phase II study to determine the efficacy of a drug, the protocol will require that the same radiographic studies done at baseline be repeated at prescribed intervals. Let us assume that the study treatment is a weekly infusion of Drug A and a cycle is 3 weeks in duration. The study procedures then might require that repeat scanning **(restaging)** be done every 6 weeks or at the end of two cycles of therapy.

Assessing the results of restaging is clearly defined in the study procedures. Typically, in oncology studies, there are five possible scenarios:

1. Complete response
2. Partial response
3. Minor response
4. Stable disease
5. Progressive disease

A *complete response* means that all disease that was seen on the baseline scans has disappeared and no new disease has developed. Each protocol dictates the exact parameters to measure other types of response. One typical criterion would define *partial response* as 50% or greater reduction in the size of the baseline tumors without development of new disease. *Minor response* often is considered a reduction of between 25% and 50% in the size of the tumors from baseline. *Stable disease* may allow up to 25% growth of the tumors, no change, or reduction of less than 25%. *Progressive disease* would be defined as overall disease growth of greater than 25%. In all cases, the appearance of a new tumor or lesion would be considered progressive disease regardless of changes in the existing tumors.

■ Calculating the Numbers

In order to define the numbers needed to calculate the percentages, many treatment centers use the Southwest Oncology Group (SWOG) Response Criteria (1999). Tumors with clearly defined margins can be measured by (1) medical photography (skin or oral lesions) or plain x-ray, with at least one diameter 0.5 centimeters or greater (bone lesions not included), or (2) CT, MRI, or other imaging study, or (3) palpation, with both diameters 2 centimeters or greater (1). Typically, discrete tumor measurements are taken in 2 dimensions, called **bidimensional measurements.** Each tumor is calculated by multiplying the two dimensions; the sum is that tumor's mass. The mass of each tumor is added to determine the patient's **total tumor burden.** A report might read as follows:

Lesion #	Site	Measurement
1	Right lobe of liver	2 cm × 1.5 cm
2	Left lobe of liver	3 cm × 2.1 cm

The tumor mass of lesion #1 is 3 cm.
The tumor mass of lesion #2 is 6.3 cm.
The total tumor burden is 9.3 cm.

Recently, in an effort to better define responses, SWOG has developed new criteria called Response Evaluation Criteria in Solid Tumors (RECIST). The system provides for a combination assessment of all existing lesions, characterized by target lesions that are measured, and non-target lesions, to extrapolate an overall response to treatment. Target lesions will be selected on the basis of their size (lesions with the longest diameter [LD]) and their suitability for accurate repetitive measurements. A sum of the LD for all target lesions will be calculated and reported as the baseline LD at the beginning of a patient's participation in a clinical trial. Restaging will require the measurement of the LD of the same target lesions for determination of response. This system defines response using slightly different percentages (20% growth = progressive disease and 30% reduction = partial response) than the bidimensional measurement criteria (2).

If lesions are not discrete enough to yield exact measurements, the disease will be considered **evaluable disease** only rather than measurable. For example, in broncheoalveolar lung cancer, disease is typically seen as a thickening in the lungs. In restaging scans, radiologists will often report the status of the disease as stable, improved or worsening. In this case the determination of response to therapy is less definitive and relies on the judgment of the physician.

Each study will define its own response criteria. Some will allow for more growth and still call it stable disease; some will be less. One reason why stable disease parameters allow for any growth at all is the technical limitations of CT scanning. During a CT scan, the machine takes pictures of the patient's body at certain intervals (cuts), for example, every 8 mm. Assuming that a tumor is round (which is rarely the case), a cut near the top of the tumor during the baseline scan might yield a measurement of 1 cm. However, at follow-up scan, the cut

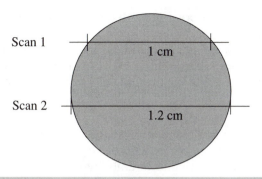

Scan 1	1 cm
Scan 2	1.2 cm

Figure 5-1 Comparison of scan measurements

might be made through the middle of the tumor. Even if the tumor did not grow, the measurement could be 1.2 cm, which would be considered a 20% growth (Fig. 5-1).

■ Adverse Events

Understanding the side effects of a new drug is an important outcome of a study. Anything the patient experiences after starting to take the study drug is called an **adverse event** and must be recorded in the study data. In order to define this information, a patient's symptoms at the time of enrollment must be clearly understood and documented. The patient's role in gathering information about adverse events is extremely important. As significant as the event itself may be, its causality or relationship to the study drug is equally important. For example, if a patient reports a headache the day after receiving the study drug, a study coordinator must know the following information:

- What was the time relationship between the onset of the headache and the receipt of the drug?
- What was the duration of the headache?
- Was any medication taken for the headache?
- Did the headache respond to medication?

Some studies will provide a diary for patients to record this information, but many do not. Therefore, a patient may be well advised to keep a journal so these details can be clearly recorded. It is important to advise the study coordinator of any other circumstances surrounding the new symptom. For example, if the patient banged his or her head getting into the car after treatment, that might have a significant impact on **causality.**

Adverse events are graded according to severity as mild, moderate, severe, and life-threatening. There are highly detailed universal criteria for grading events. Using the example of a headache, the criteria reads as follows:

Grade 1: mild pain not interfering with functioning

Grade 2: moderate pain, where pain or analgesics interfere with function but not with activities of daily living

Grade 3: severe pain, where pain or analgesics severely interfere with activities of daily living

Grade 4: disabling (3)

A **serious adverse event** is an occurrence that results in a hospitalization, causes significant disability, is life-threatening (patient is in immediate risk of death), or results in death. Determining causality and promptly reporting the event to the sponsor is paramount. If the serious adverse event is determined to be related or possibly related to the study drug, the sponsor must file a report (called a *MedWatch*) to the FDA and to all physicians who are currently using or have used that particular drug in studies.

Sometimes, a patient who is participating in a clinical trial continues to see the primary physician or primary oncologist who is closer to home. For that reason, if a physician other than the study physician institutes a treatment or hospitalizes a patient, it is very important that the study coordinator or study physician be informed in a timely manner. The safety of other patients receiving the study drug may be at stake.

■ Phases of Clinical Trials

Clinical trials that are designed to study drugs or treatments are conducted in four phases, designated I through IV.

Phase I

A phase I study answers questions of safety:

What is the safe dose of the drug?

What are the side effects?

How is the drug metabolized?

From the patient's perspective, it is important to understand that these are the most basic of questions. Phase I is the first time the drug is being tested in humans. What is known about the drug is only from the animal studies. No information about the effective dose or the side effects in humans is yet known.

The success of the drug in animal studies may not translate to humans. No matter how optimistic the investigators are about the drug, no one knows if the drug is safe in humans or if it will have any efficacy. No matter how much media attention this drug or other drugs like it have received, there are still no human data.

The most frequently asked question when discussing a phase I study is, "Does it work?" The answer must always be, "I don't know." Any other answer is irresponsible. Why then would a patient consent to participation in a phase I trial? For many patients, all known therapy has been exhausted and they may not be eligible for phase II or III trials. If they want to have treatment, a phase I clinical trial may be the only possibility. Some patients will say that they have nothing to lose and perhaps something to gain. Others will say that even if the treatment will not help them, perhaps the information gleaned from the study will contribute to future generations. Clearly, participation in a phase I study is a value judgment.

Phase I trials are always single agent studies, meaning only the study drug is given to patients. Because the objective of a phase I study is to define the side-effect profile of the drug, combining it with other drugs is not allowed. When two or more drugs are used in combination, there could be side effects caused by drug–drug interactions. If a side effect is seen in such a situation, how will the investigator know if the side effect is related to the study drug, the other drug, or the combination thereof? Therefore, the safe dose and the side-effect profile must be defined before the drug can go onto phase II clinical trials or be combined with other drugs.

The number of patients who will participate in a phase I trial is difficult to define at the outset of the study. The typical design is for three patients to be given the drug at the starting dose determined from the preclinical trials (see discussion about lethal dose in animals). If all three patients complete a cycle (often 3 to 4 weeks) taking the drug without unacceptable side effects, the dose is escalated by a predetermined percentage, and three more patients will take the drug at the new, higher dose.

The dose escalation scheme continues in that fashion until one patient experiences an unacceptable side effect (toxicity). An unacceptable side effect could be an abnormal value on a blood test or vomiting or diarrhea that does not respond to treatment. It is important to understand that most toxicities will reverse when the drug is stopped.

If one of the three patients in a particular dose group **(cohort)** experiences an unacceptable toxicity, the investigator must decide if the symptom is related to the study drug, the patient's disease, or some totally unrelated illness (for example, the flu). To better define the situation, three more patients are enrolled at the same dose. After six patients have received the drug at that dose level, if only one patient has demonstrated that particular symptom, the dose level is determined to be safe and dose escalation resumes. However, if two of the six patients demonstrate the same toxicity, then it is presumed that further escalation of the dose could cause serious injury to a patient and the study is stopped. The toxicity that caused the study to stop is called the **dose-limiting toxicity (DLT).** The dose that preceded the DLT is then considered the safe dose and is declared the **maximum tolerated dose (MTD),** the dose that can be given to humans without unacceptable toxicity.

Predicting how many patients will participate in a phase I study or exactly when each cohort will begin is very difficult. It is possible that the DLT may be determined after only 15 patients, or it may not be found until 70 patients have taken the drug. If anywhere along the way there are concerns about the safety of the drug, the study may be stopped while the physicians and scientists try to get a clearer understanding of the situation. Patient safety is the foremost concern.

Patients often ask the question about efficacy in a phase I study. Typically, patients with a variety of different diagnoses are included in a phase I study. For example, in a 30-patient study, there could be ten different diagnoses represented. If, for example, three of those 30 patients have lung cancer and two of them show a response (meaning that their tumors got smaller while taking the drug), can the conclusion be drawn that the study drug works in lung cancer? Certainly not! The statisticians will say that the sample is too small. Such a finding has absolutely no statistical significance. The finding may, however, suggest that further testing of the drug in lung cancer is indicated and a phase II study will be designed.

Phase II

A phase II clinical trial answers the question of efficacy. Does this drug work? Not every drug will work in every cancer. Most drugs will be efficacious in just a few diseases. The decision about which diseases to test in a phase II study is determined by information from the testing done on cell lines in the preclinical work and possibly by patients who may have shown a response in the phase I trials.

Typically, phase II studies will include a homogeneous group of patients. For example, the study may be designed for lung cancer patients who have metastatic disease (disease outside the lungs) and have not had prior treatment. The sponsor makes that decision, not the investigator. No matter how insistent a colon cancer patient may be about receiving the drug, if the study is for lung cancer patients, then only lung cancer patients can participate.

In a phase II study, all of the patients receive the study drug at the same dose on the same schedule, for example, weekly dosing. Recall the purpose of the study is to determine efficacy. Therefore, 30 patients with untreated lung cancer are given Drug A at 100 mg. At a prescribed interval, for example, 8 weeks, the patient is tested and the results are compared to the results of tests done prior to the treatment. If six patients show a reduction in the size of their tumors, then Drug A is said to have 20% efficacy (6/30 patients) in patients with untreated lung cancer.

Phase I/II

After the safe dose of a drug is determined in a phase I study, the sponsor may choose to study the new drug in combination with an established, FDA-approved drug. In this situation, the safe dose of each drug as a single agent is known; however, there is a possibility of new side effects caused by the combination of the drugs (drug–drug interactions). The starting dose of one or both of the drugs will be lower than the safe dose of the drug when used as a single agent. For example, if Drug A's (the new drug) safe dose is 100 mg and Drug B's (the established drug) safe dose is 200 mg, the study may begin with Drug A given at 50 mg and Drug B at 150 mg. After three patients are safely treated at those doses, the dose of one drug will be escalated while the other remains constant. For example, for the next cohort (group of three patients), Drug A's dose will be 75 mg while Drug B's dose remains 150 mg. If that dose is determined to be safe, the next cohort will be treated with Drug A at 75 mg and Drug B's dose escalated to 175 mg. Pharmacokinetics (special blood tests to determine drug levels) are done at each new dose level to determine if one drug is potentiating the other, causing higher drug levels than seen in the earlier studies.

The objectives of a phase I/II study are not only finding the safe dose, but also determining the efficacy of the combination of the two drugs. These studies may be small (20 patients or less) and are called **pilot studies.** The purpose of a pilot study is to establish the safety and potential efficacy of the combination to move into larger phase III studies and FDA approval.

Interim Analysis

Sometimes an **interim analysis** will be conducted during a phase II study. Typically, an interim analysis will be done after one-half of the anticipated enrollment has been achieved. For example, in a study designed to enroll 40 patients, enrollment will be suspended after 20 patients have started the study medication. The purpose of the analysis is to determine if any of the first 20 patients will have a response to the study medication. If 20 patients are restaged and not one patient demonstrates a response, the study will be terminated for lack of efficacy. However, if even one patient has a response, then the study will resume accrual and complete the anticipated 40-patient enrollment.

An interim analysis can also be conducted for safety reasons during any phase of clinical testing. For example, if several patients experience a similar serious and unexpected toxicity, enrollment will be suspended in order to perform a careful review of the data to determine if the drug is safe for administration in humans.

Phase III

Phase III studies are large multicenter studies in which hundreds of patients are enrolled. The purpose is to compare a new treatment with at least one other existing effective therapy. Each treatment being tested in the trial is called a **study arm.** Patients who enroll in the trial are **randomized,** that is, randomly assigned to one of the study arms. Patients do not have a choice of which arm or treatment they will receive.

As an example, let us review a study completed in 1999 to compare two existing treatments for colorectal cancer with a new treatment. For 40 years, the drug 5-fluorouracil (5-FU) was used to treat colorectal cancer. Many different modulations (methods of delivery) of 5-FU elicited changes in the side-effect profile but no difference in survival (4). Calcium leucovorin, a mineral, when given with 5-FU was found to improve the response rate, but did not improve survival. Because of the improvement in response, leucovorin was added to 5-FU and the combination became the standard of care (5).

In 1998, a new drug called irinotecan (Camptosar) was found to have approximately 15% efficacy against colon cancer. The FDA approved it as a single agent for the treatment of colorectal cancer in patients who had failed 5-FU and leucovorin therapy (second-line therapy) (6).

However, the sponsors of irinotecan thought that the drug might be just as effective as 5-FU and leucovorin as a first-line therapy (in patients who had not received other therapy). Therefore, they designed a study that had three study arms:

- Arm A: 5-FU and leucovorin alone
- Arm B: irinotecan alone
- Arm C: 5-FU, leucovorin, and irinotecan in combination

Many physicians were skeptical because diarrhea was a side effect associated with both 5-FU and irinotecan, and they feared that the combination of those drugs would cause uncontrollable diarrhea.

Patients who enrolled in the study were randomized to receive one of the three treatments. It is important to understand that Arms A and B both were known to be effective therapies for colorectal cancer; therefore, every patient was receiving effective treatment. The question was whether one therapy was more effective than the others.

At the conclusion of the study, it was determined that patients receiving the combination of all three drugs had a longer interval without progression of the disease and a longer time to survival (patients lived longer) than either of the other two arms (7,8). The incidence of diarrhea with the combination therapy was less than 10% greater than with 5-FU and leucovorin alone and was well controlled with aggressive use of loperamide, a common over-the-counter drug used for diarrhea. The data were presented to the FDA in April 2000, and the combination therapy received FDA approval as first-line therapy.

In some two-arm studies, the group of patients receiving the standard of care may be called the **control arm.** The group of patients receiving the new treatment will be called the **treatment arm.**

Phase IV

Phase IV studies are conducted after a drug has received FDA approval and is commercially available. These studies generally are done to determine other uses for the drug *(off-label uses)* and to further assess side effects (10).

Preventative Studies

Clinical trials sometimes are conducted to evaluate the potential of people to develop cancer. For example, a group of healthy volunteers may be recruited to participate in a study to define the effect of diet on the development of breast cancer. Typically, these are randomized studies in which women are assigned to a specific group. Group A may eat diets that have less than 20% fat content; group B may eat a diet with at least 40% fat content. These studies often continue over a long time, perhaps several decades, and are called *longitudinal studies.* The final analysis of the data is expected to determine if a low-fat diet will positively impact the overall incidence of breast cancer.

Studies of Drugs that Control Symptoms

Other studies may be designed to look at drugs that have the potential to impact symptoms associated with cancer treatment. The experimental drugs could be used to treat nausea, vomiting, diarrhea, fatigue, or low blood counts as an example. These studies frequently are as important as studies defining new therapies, because the control of symptoms may allow patients to take or continue treatment that would otherwise be discontinued because the patient's side effects are a limiting factor.

Patients typically are not allowed to participate in more than one experimental therapy at the same time. The concern is the possibility of interactions between the two experimental drugs, called *drug–drug interactions.* If there were some unexpected symptom, it would be impossible to determine which drug was causing the problem or whether it was the combination of the two drugs that was the problem. Therefore, if a patient is enrolled in a study with a drug to control nausea, he or she would not be eligible for a study of an experimental drug to treat the cancer. Clearly, most patients would choose to participate in a study that focuses on treatment rather than on symptom control if the situation arises.

Quality-of-Life Questionnaires

In many phase III studies, a **quality-of-life questionnaire** is part of the study procedures. Patients are asked to complete a questionnaire before beginning to take the drug and then again at certain intervals during treatment, including when the patient stops treatment. The questions typically deal with the patients' activities, pain level, and perception of subjective things such as fatigue. Although a new treatment may show very little objective improvement in the time to response or survival, it may improve the patient's quality of life. In cancer patients, that may be a significant finding and something the FDA takes into consideration when analyzing a drug for approval.

Blinded Studies

Sometimes, a study is **blinded,** meaning only the pharmacist who prepares the drug knows which treatment the patient is receiving. The purpose of blinding a study is to avoid bias. At times, patients will tell the study coordinator that the minute they received the new drug, they began to feel better. The coordinator, and sometimes the patient, knows that the drug has not yet had an opportunity to work. This is known as the *Hawthorne Effect* (see the explanation below). The sponsor who designs a blinded study may believe that investigators and study coordinators, if they know which treatment the patient is receiving, could be influenced in the way they interpret and record their observations.

The Hawthorne Studies

Beginning in 1924, researchers sponsored by the National Academy of Sciences studied the effects of lighting on worker productivity at the Hawthorne Works of the Western Electric Company, near Chicago. The early results were puzzling because regardless of whether the researchers increased or decreased the lighting, the workers' productivity either remained constant or exceeded normal output. Even if the lighting was so low that the workers could barely see what they were doing, the results remained the same. Following observations and interviews, the researchers concluded that the effect was due to the attention that the workers were getting and not due to changes in working conditions. This phenomenon was later termed the "Hawthorne Effect" (9).

Some randomized, blinded studies may use a **placebo** (a drug without any therapeutic intent) as a control arm. In these studies, patients on both arms will receive what appears to be the same treatment, for example, an intravenous infusion over 1 hour, but one group of patients will receive just the intravenous fluid without any drug in it.

These studies usually are done in a disease where no effective treatment is known. The purpose of the study is to determine if a given treatment has any benefit over no active treatment for the disease. No treatment in cancer is typically called **best supportive care,** meaning the patient's symptoms are treated as they arise. When considering participation in a blinded study, it is important to ask if one arm is a placebo.

In some studies, treatment **cross-over** is allowed. Take the case of a patient who enrolls in a blinded study and is assigned to the placebo arm. Typically, at the end of the assessment period (usually 4 to 6 weeks), the patient receiving the placebo will be allowed to cross over to the treatment arm and then begin to receive the study medication. Sometimes cross-over is allowed in other randomized studies. When planning to enroll in a randomized study, ask if cross-over is allowed.

■ References

1. *Southwest Oncology Group Clinical Research Manual* (1999). Vol I, Chapters 7-2-7-11.
2. Therasse, P., Arbuck, SG, Eisenhauer, EA, et al. New guidelines to evaluate the response to treatment in solid tumors. *Journal of the National Cancer Institute* 2000;92(3):205–216.
3. CTC version 2.0, revised March 23, 1998.
4. Leichman CG, Fleming TR, Muggia FM, et al. Phase II study of fluorouracil and its modulation in advanced colorectal cancer: a Southwest Oncology Group study. *J Clin Oncol* 1995;13:1303–1311.
5. Treatment of advanced colorectal cancer. Available at *http://intouch .cancernetwork.com/CanMed/CH121/121-18.htm*. Accessed August 6, 2000.
6. Von Hoff DD, Rothenberg ML, Pitot HC, et al. Irinotecan (CPT-11) therapy for patients with previously treated metastatic colorectal cancer (CRC): overall results of FDA-reviewed pivotal U.S. clinical trials. *Proc Am Soc Clin Oncol* 1997;16:abst 803,228a.
7. Saltz LB, Douillard J, Pirotta N, et al. Combined analysis of two phase III randomized trials comparing irinotecan (C), fluorouracil (F), leucovorin (L) vs. F alone as first-line therapy of previously untreated metastatic colorectal cancer (MCRC). *Proc Am Soc Clin Oncol* 2000;19:abst 938,242a.
8. Saltz LB, Cox JV, Blanke C, et al. Irinotecan plus fluorouracil and leucovorin for metastatic colorectal cancer. *N Engl J Med* 2000;343:905–914.
9. Fisher D. *Communication in organizations,* 2nd ed. Minneapolis/St. Paul: West Publishing Company, 1983:69–70.
10. Mulay M. *Step-by-step guide to clinical trials.* Sudbury, MA: Jones and Bartlett, 2001:9–10.

CHAPTER 6

The Business of Clinical Research

■ The Approval Process

Once the protocol is written and approved, the sponsor forwards it to the participating medical centers. The number of patients expected to be enrolled typically dictates the number of sites that will participate in each study. For example, a phase I study with an anticipated enrollment of 30 patients may be conducted at only one or two centers. However, a phase III study with a projected enrollment of 700 may be conducted at 50 different centers. Regardless of the number of centers, each center must follow the same process of approval by its individual **institutional review board (IRB).**

■ History of the Protection of Human Subjects

In 1963, a New York hospital set out to study immune response to cancer. Some elderly, ill, and feeble patients were injected with cancer cells. They were told that their resistance was being measured; they were not told they were being injected with cancer cells. Fortunately, the project was stopped soon after it began, and none of the patients developed cancer (1). The Nazi experiments on Jewish prisoners during World War II are well-documented atrocities. To develop a vaccine for typhoid fever, prisoners were injected with blood from infected patients. As a result of these and other violations of human rights, the need to protect subjects of research was evident. See Chapter 7 for more information on this subject.

■ Development of the Informed Consent Process

The Kefauver-Harris Amendments to the Food, Drug, and Cosmetic Act was passed in 1962. It was the first law that required research subjects to give **informed consent** before they could be treated with an experimental drug. The Act only required that verbal consent be given and documented in the patient's chart (1).

In 1966, the Public Health Service (PHS) required that for a study to receive PHS funding, subjects must be told about the benefits, risks, and purpose of the research. However, it was not until 1967 that the United States Food and Drug Administration (FDA) policy statement required that the consent be obtained in writing (1).

The informed consent is discussed in detail in Chapter 7.

■ Birth of Institutional Review Boards

In 1976, the FDA issued regulations requiring that a committee review all studies using institutionalized subjects. The regulations were refined further in 1981 to require that all studies involving humans must be reviewed and approved by an Institutional Review Board (IRB) in order to receive an FDA permit (1).

Typically, an IRB consists of at least five people of varying backgrounds. Some may have training or background in research areas; others may represent other disciplines. For example, a committee may consist of one or more of the following: physicians who practice in the clinical area, scientists who work in medical research, pharmacists, and social workers. Racial, ethnic, and other interests may be represented by at least one member from a nonscientific background, generally a lawyer or a member of the clergy. At least one member of the IRB must not be affiliated with the research institution (1).

The purpose of an IRB is to protect the rights of individuals who enroll in clinical trials. The inception is steeped in history (see Chapter 7 for more information on the history and development of laws and agencies to protect a patient's rights).

■ The IRB and the Patient

Institutional review boards vary from institution to institution, and the filing procedures also vary widely. Some IRBs may be informal, requiring a minimal amount of paperwork; others require many forms and rigorous review of the information. Regardless of the actual procedures, every IRB reviews every protocol and its informed consent before patients can be enrolled. In many institutions, this is a very intense process designed to provide safe and ethical treatment of human subjects.

The IRB review ensures that

- Risks to participants are minimized. Study procedures are consistent with **Good Clinical Practice (GCP)** guidelines and do not expose patients to unnecessary risks.
- Informed consent is obtained and documented from each participant or his or her legal representative.
- Patient selection is fair and equitable, and there are safeguards to protect those who are not able to look out for their own interests, such as mentally retarded patients.
- Risks to participants are reasonable in relation to the expected benefits and the importance of the knowledge that may be gained.
- The participant's privacy is protected and provisions are in place to maintain data confidentiality (2).

The entire process of IRB approval may take from a few weeks to several months. After all of the forms are completed, the protocol is submitted and placed in a queue. After the initial review, a letter is sent to the principal investigator outlining questions and concerns. If there is concern that the design of the protocol will not prove the objectives of the study, the sponsor may need to revise the protocol or write a letter of explanation to the IRB. When the IRB's concerns are satisfied, then approval will be granted. If patients are waiting for approval to begin the study, the wait can seem interminable.

Patients should feel assured that the IRB is diligently working on their behalf. The informed consent that a patient signs prior to starting any study procedures will tell him or her how to contact the institution's IRB should any questions or concerns arise.

Even after a study is initiated, the IRB keeps a close watch on the ongoing trial. Every serious adverse event (SAE) report must be filed with the IRB. If there is concern that the SAE is related to the study drug, the protocol and consent will be amended to ensure that all participants are informed of the new development. MedWatches (reports of serious adverse events believed to be related to the study drug) also are filed with the IRB. Every study must be renewed on a yearly basis, with an accompanying annual report that summarizes the enrollment and safety data over the course of the past year.

Every physician who is an investigator or **co-investigator** in a study must file a financial disclosure statement with the IRB. The purpose is to ensure that the results of the study could not financially benefit a physician and, therefore, bias the patient selection for participation or color the interpretation of the information.

■ Budgetary Issues

The execution of a clinical trial is a contractual agreement between the sponsor and the principal investigator. Therefore, a budget and a contract must be agreed to and signed by both parties prior to enrolling patients. Many people are involved in the successful execution of a protocol, and every detail is important.

When patients participate in a clinical trial, the patient's insurance company typically pays the costs of routine patient care. The premise is that these are costs that patients would incur for any treatment for their disease. In today's environment of managed care, routine has become a complicated concept. This will be discussed in more detail in Chapter 9. The costs of any procedures in excess of routine patient care, such as laboratory tests or radiographic examinations, and the experimental treatment itself, are the responsibility of the sponsor. The sponsor also is expected to pay for the time spent by the principal investigator, the study coordinator, and the data manager to care for the patients and collect and record the data.

The principal investigator prepares a budget that outlines the cost of all procedures beyond the routine items. In some institutions, the budget proposal must be reviewed by a budget committee to ensure that all of the institution's costs are adequately covered.

Once the budget has been approved at the institution level, it is sent to the sponsor for approval. Frequently, a budget committee also exists at the sponsoring company. Studies being done at multiple sites might have budgets that vary considerably because of the differences of doing business in different parts of the country or world.

■ The Contract

Once the budget is agreed to, the **contract** must be negotiated. The contract specifies that the study will be conducted under Good

Clinical Practice (GCP) guidelines, establishes the payment schedule, and assigns the rights to publish the findings of the research. The contract includes definitions of indemnification and liability as well as noncompete clauses, which prohibits the parties signing the contract from participating in trials that compete with this study (3).

Legal counsel for both the sponsor and the medical center may have different opinions about any or all of the clauses contained in the contract. In large medical centers affiliated with a statewide system, many of the issues are dictated by a board of regents that oversees all university contracts. This too is a process that can take several weeks to resolve.

■ Other Time-Consuming Details

Once the budget and the contract are signed, sealed, and delivered, a site initiation is scheduled. During a site initiation, the sponsor sends representatives to the medical center to review the protocol and related procedures with study personnel. They will visit the clinic and treatment area as well as the pharmacy where the drug will be dispensed. They will observe the place where the drug will be stored to ensure that it will be stored under proper conditions. They review drug accountability procedures with the chief pharmacist to be certain that all of the drug received and dispensed will be appropriately accounted for.

Let's review:

- IRB approval
- Budget
- Contract
- Site initiation

Once all these requirements are met, the sponsor will ship the drug to the medical center. The final step in preparation for enrolling patients is an inservice to the nursing staff that will be administering the drug. Nurses are responsible for the patients they treat and, therefore, must have all available information on a new drug. They will want to know exactly how the drug is given and what potential side effects they might see. The treatment nurses are an important link in the research continuum, and their education about the protocol procedures is paramount to the success of the study.

■ These Issues and the Patient

It may seem that none of these issues directly impacts the participants in a study. However, the time impact can be significant. For patients anxious to begin an experimental treatment, the waiting may be very difficult. Perhaps understanding that most of these procedures are done to ensure patient safety will make the waiting a little more tolerable.

■ References

1. Thompson RC. Protecting "human guinea pigs." FDA consumer special report. Available at *http://www.fda.gov/fdac/special/newdrug/guinea.html.* Accessed November 29, 2000.
2. International Conference on Harmonisation. Good clinical practice: consolidated guideline: notice of availability. *Federal Register* 1997;62:90.
3. Mulay M. *Step-by-step guide to clinical trials.* Sudbury, MA: Jones and Bartlett Publishers, 2001:45.

CHAPTER 7

The Patient's Rights

Every person within the health care system must be an informed participant in his or her own medical care. The days of "Whatever the doctor says is OK with me" are gone. Understanding the diagnosis and treatment are important factors in the care a patient receives.

Participation in a clinical trial does not make a patient a guinea pig. Quite the contrary! The patient is, in fact, a research subject who receives good medical care while receiving an experimental therapy. Participation in clinical trials is actually associated with higher survival rates than those patients who are treated conventionally (1). The reason for this is unclear. It may be that patients receive a more effective treatment or that patients are treated in a more disciplined way that translates to better overall treatment (2). There are many safeguards in place to ensure the patient's rights are protected; however, the responsibility of a patient to understand the process and be informed cannot be overemphasized.

■ The History of Legislation

A dark history spurred the development and adoption of legislation to protect those who participate in clinical trials. The history is presented here to inform potential participants about past transgressions and emphasizes the need to be informed.

In the late 1900s, great industries began to arise. Government supported the growth of business, and any social change to benefit that growth was acceptable. By the turn of the century, it was clear that legislation was needed to safeguard the interests of citizens worldwide. In 1906, Upton Sinclair published his now classic novel, *The Jungle*, which exposed unsanitary meat handling in Chicago's slaughterhouses (3). Although seen as propaganda at the time, the book spurred passage of the Food and Drug Law of 1906. Further legislation came in response to an elixir of sulfanilamide, marketed by the Massengill Drug Company, that killed 107 people. The Food, Drug, and Cosmetic Drug Act of 1938 was the first law to require that companies establish *drug safety* prior to marketing a compound.

The Declaration of Helsinki was issued in Finland in 1961 (4). The declaration, which is internationally recognized as a worldwide standard in clinical trials, addresses standards for medical personnel in research with human subjects. The United States Public Health Service mandated use of Institutional Review Boards (IRBs) and issued regulations for informed consent involving human research subjects in 1966. Other amendments included requirements for use of accurate and ethical advertising to recruit subjects.

■ The History of Ethical Guidelines

During World War II, research atrocities were performed on prisoners of war. In 1946, during the Nuremberg trials, 23 physicians were tried for their wartime activities. As a result, the **Nuremberg Code** was issued in 1947 as the first internationally recognized code of research ethics. Unfortunately, many researchers did not understand how this code applied to their research (5).

In 1962, following the thalidomide disaster in which more than 300 babies were born with anomalies from a drug given to their mothers for nausea, the Kefauver-Harris Amendments to the Food, Drug, and Cosmetic Act were passed. They required companies to establish the efficacy of their products as well as adhere to new requirements with regards to purity and safety before making the products available to the public (6).

In an address to Congress in 1962, President John F. Kennedy, proclaimed the Consumer Bill of Rights. This proclamation included the rights to safety, to be informed, to choose, and to be heard. In many states, a patient's bill of rights is attached to every informed consent form (ICF) (7).

The ethics of clinical trials again came into unfavorable focus when, in 1972, an account of the Tuskegee Syphilis Study sparked public outrage. In 1932, the U.S. Public Health Service began a study of syphilis in black men in the small rural town of Tuskegee, Alabama. The purpose of the study was to determine the natural course of syphilis in adult black men. The study group included 400 men with untreated syphilis. The control group included 200 men without syphilis. Even though penicillin was then known to be an effective treatment for syphilis, the men were not treated. In fact, deliberate steps were taken to keep the subjects from receiving treatment.

It was determined that information had been withheld from study participants. Many did not understand the purpose of the study, and some did not realize they were participating in a study. Reports of the study were published as early as 1936, but no action was taken to stop the study. Even as late as 1969, the Center for Disease Control believed that the study should continue. Finally, after the public outrage of 1972, the Department of Health, Education, and Welfare stopped the study (8). These accounts are some of the worst-case scenarios of disregard for the rights and welfare of patients participating in clinical trials. Because of these and other ethically questionable situations, the ethics of clinical research became an arena of suspicion and mistrust. As a result, in 1974, The National Commission for the Protection of Human Subjects of Biomedical and Behavioral Research was established. It examined the issue of human experimentation and explored its ethical and human rights implications. The commission's findings and recommendations were published in 1978 in *The Belmont Report: Ethical Principles and Guidelines for the Protection of Human Subjects*, which established stricter guidelines for the information provided to research subjects (8).

The principles outlined in *The Belmont Report* now govern all research supported by the U.S. government through its regulatory agency, the U.S. Food and Drug Administration (FDA). The principles are

- Respect for persons
- Beneficence
- Justice

Respect for persons acknowledges the dignity and freedom of every person and requires that each research subject give informed consent before participating in a clinical trial. *Beneficence* requires that researchers maximize benefits and minimize risks, and that there must be a reasonable balance between risks and benefits. And finally, *justice* requires that selection and recruitment of research subjects be equitable and their treatment be fair.

The goal is to promote greater respect for an individual's autonomy and give greater attention to beneficence and justice for all humans involved in clinical trials. The report addressed the need for documentation of the risks versus benefits of a clinical trial in the ICF and to set guidelines for special protection of children and the mentally ill.

In the early 1980s, the regulations for the conduct of research with humans were revised and published as the *Title 45 Code of Federal Regulations Part 46, Protection of Human Subjects (45CFR46)* (9).

■ Good Clinical Practice Guidelines

All clinical trials must be conducted within Good Clinical Practice (GCP) guidelines. Good Clinical Practice guidelines is an international ethical and scientific quality standard for designing, conducting, recording, and reporting clinical trials that involve the participation of human subjects. The origin of this guideline is the Declaration of Helsinki (1961); GCP provides public assurance that the rights, safety, and well-being of participants in clinical trials are protected. The objective of GCP guidelines is to provide a unified standard for the European Union (EU), Japan, and the United States in order to facilitate the mutual acceptance of clinical data by the regulatory authorities in those jurisdictions. The latest update of these guidelines was published in May 1997 as a result of the **International Conference on Harmonisation (ICH).**

■ United States Food and Drug Administration

The FDA is a part of the U.S. Department of Health and Human Service. Its history dates back to 1862, when President Lincoln established the Bureau of Chemistry. Evolving through several names and departments, its purview includes all aspects of manufacturing and marketing of both prescription and over-the-counter drugs. In 1937, the agency established the Code of Federal Regulations (CFR), which codifies its regulations and sets guidelines for many aspects of clinical trials (10).

In addition to monitoring food and drugs, the FDA also provides resources for the public. A new service called *Oncology Tools* is being offered on the Internet and can be found at *www.fda.gov/cder/cancer/ index.htm.* By accessing this web site, a patient can find information about approved oncology drugs, disease summaries, oncology reference tools, a patient liaison program, and much more. This is currently a pilot project, and the FDA is anxious for comments by users (11).

■ Informed Consent

See Chapter 7 for information on the history of informed consent.

When an IRB places its stamp of approval on a protocol, it also approves the ICF, the document a patient signs as an agreement to participate in a clinical trial.

Informed consent has been a hot topic for years and will likely always be so. Volumes have been written about informed consent, the patient's right to know, and the patient's bill of rights, among others. Indeed, each of these issues is extremely important. How much detail an informed consent must include often is driven by an institution's IRB. For example, at some institutions, it does not suffice to say that the patient will have certain blood tests; instead, the amount of blood to be drawn must be stated in layman's terms, that is, in teaspoons or tablespoons.

Clarity of Language

The most important issue about writing an informed consent is that it must be in language that all patients can understand. Well-informed participants should not be offended if the language seems elementary; it is intended to be written at an eighth-grade reading level. For example, the ICF will describe intravenous as "through a needle in your vein."

Level of Detail

Concerns about liability and the patient's right to know have prompted consent forms that are 10 to 20 pages long. Undoubtedly, there will always be patients who absorb every word and still want more information, as well as patients who are overwhelmed just look-ing at a document that looks that formal. The FDA guidelines of 1995 allow the use of shorter consent forms, but most IRBs continue to advocate detailed consent forms to guarantee that participants are fully informed.

Need for Translation

The FDA has mandated that every participant in a clinical trial must receive a copy of the informed consent in his or her native language. Because patients from varied ethnic backgrounds participate in clinical trials, it is impossible to accurately anticipate the need for consent forms in all possible translations. Although a patient may be consented with a translator present, he or she also must receive a translated copy of the consent form to sign.

Late Details and Revisions

During the course of a clinical trial, new information may arise. For example, some patients may experience an unanticipated cough that may be related to the drug. Such information is communicated to the patients currently in the trial as soon as it is known, and then a revised consent form must be written. The revised consent is again sent for approval by the IRB. Once approved, all of the patients in the study must be reconsented; they must sign the new consent. Depending on the length of time a patient is on a specific trial, he or she may sign several consents.

Understanding the Informed Consent Form

Most consents will address the following areas of importance.

Purpose of the Study

This information describes why the protocol has been designed and what it expects to prove. As a patient, understanding the purpose of the study will help to decide if this trial is appropriate to meet his or her needs.

Procedures Involved in Participating in the Study

This section will identify, step by step, what is involved from the first screening visit through the follow-up visit, after participation in the study has been completed. This section will include information about all blood tests, electrocardiograms, computerized tomography scans, physical examinations, and anything else the patient will be asked to undergo during the course of the study and give a sense of the time commitment required.

Potential Risks and Discomforts

All possible side effects will be outlined in this section. The information is gleaned from previous animal and human trials, if applicable. In addition to describing what is known about the drug, the ICF will state that previously unknown side effects may occur, even death. This statement is not intended to frighten the patient, but all possible side effects are required to be stated.

The risk of pregnancy is discussed, with the statement that patients of childbearing potential also must agree to use adequate methods of contraception because the effects of the drug(s) on unborn fetuses are not known.

Potential Benefits

This is usually a brief statement of what benefits have already been seen in animal and/or human trials, with a caveat that the drug(s) may be of no benefit at all to the participants. A statement about the potential contribution of participation to other people or future research typically is made here.

No one can guarantee any benefit to the patient. Although investigators are hopeful that the drug or procedure will benefit patients, depending on the phase of the trial, there is a chance that patients may not receive any benefit at all. Ethical investigators will be sure that patients understand that premise. Although no one wants to destroy hope, patients must understand the limitations of a study.

Alternative to Participation

Other alternatives to participation in the trial are briefly discussed in this section. The options typically include

- Best supportive care (no active treatment against the cancer)
- Conventional therapy (treatment with FDA-approved drugs)
- Experimental therapy (investigational drugs other than the drug(s) involved in this study)

Compensation for Participation

Typically in cancer clinical trials, patients are not paid for participation. If there is to be payment, this section will state so, how much, and when payment will be made.

Financial Obligation

This is a section that always evokes questions. In general, the study drug, its administration, and all tests that are specifically related to the experimental nature of the study are provided or paid for by the study's sponsor. Blood tests and other procedures that are normally part of the care of a patient being treated for the particular disease can and should be billed to insurance. This will be discussed in more detail in Chapter 9.

Emergency Care and Compensation for Injury

If the patient is injured as a result of participation in the study, the sponsor is expected to pay for the patient's treatment. However, customarily there is a statement indemnifying the participating medical institution from liability. If a problem arises during the course of a clinical trial, it may be difficult initially to determine if the cause is the underlying disease or the study drug. Typically, if the drug is the source of the problem, the symptom(s) will go away when the patient stops taking the drug.

Confidentiality

This section assures patients that their identities will remain confidential. Although information about the patient's treatment and response will be shared with the sponsor, the FDA, the IRB, and the researchers participating in the study, every effort will be made to guarantee the patient's privacy. There also will be a statement about needing to obtain records of previous treatment from other institutions. This allows the study coordinator use of this page and the signature page to obtain any needed records from other institutions where the patient previously received care.

Participation and Withdrawal

This section should begin with a statement that participation in the study is **voluntary.** It will also state that a patient may withdraw consent at any time. Conditions under which continued participation is allowed are if the disease does not progress, there are no severe toxicities, the patient complies with study requirements, and the study is not discontinued. Patients should ask about continuing the treatment if they are receiving benefit from it. The information a sponsor needs about a drug probably will be gathered in the first month or two of a patient's participation. Patients should have assurance that the treatment will not be withdrawn after the needed data are gathered.

On the other hand, patients must conform with the requirements of the study to ensure their continued participation. When a study requires blood tests at particular intervals, the patients must comply to ensure continued safety. Failure to do so may result in removal from the study.

New Findings

There will be a statement that if any new information is obtained, good or bad, a patient will be informed. If a finding is significant, the informed consent will be revised and resigned by all participants.

Identification of Investigators

The principal investigator and all of the subinvestigators (other physicians participating in the trial) will be named, and their addresses, telephone numbers, and emergency numbers will be provided.

Rights of Research Subjects

Another statement about the patient's right to withdraw consent at any time is under this section. Also, the name, address, and telephone number of the IRB will be given in case patients have any questions about their rights.

Signature Page

This is a brief statement that the patient has read and understands all of the information in the consent form and acknowledges receipt of a copy of the consent. The form may provide a line for the patient's name to be printed, then a line for the signature followed by the date and time. The FDA requires that the consent be obtained prior to any screening procedures. If screening is being done on the same day consent is secured, then the time will indicate whether the FDA guideline has been met.

Although only the patient's signature is required on the consent, many institutions require that the document be countersigned by the investigator or the designee who explained the consent. Date and time should follow this signature as well.

If the patient is a minor and has a guardian, or needs a translator, then the guardian or translator also needs to sign the consent, indicating the relationship or role in the consenting process as well as the date and time of signature (12).

Ensuring the Safeguards

How does the patient know if all of these safeguards are being followed? There are several mechanisms in place to ensure that the investigator, medical institution, and sponsor follow all of the regulations and guidelines.

The sponsor monitors the conduct of the clinical trial in a variety of ways. Before the protocol is filed with the IRB, the sponsor must agree to the ICF, assuring that the clinical trial is properly represented in the document. Many of the other regulatory documents also are filed with the sponsor. During the course of the trial, the sponsor monitors the activities at the research center by reviewing the data collected on the patient. The review not only ensures that the protocol is being executed properly but that all of the data collection is true and correct. The monitor will check the regulatory documents to ensure that the IRB has been kept informed of all study activities. A visit to the pharmacy verifies that the drug is being dispensed properly and the drug accountability logs are in order.

A sponsor may decide to conduct an **audit** of a particular study to ensure that the site is following all the protocol procedures. This type of audit not only checks the data entry at the clinical site but also double-checks the work of the monitor.

Within the institution, a committee of the IRB may conduct quality assurance (QA) audits. The committee rotates their audits to monitor the conduct of various investigators. A percentage of patient charts is reviewed again to ensure that the patients have been properly consented and are being treated within the dictates of the protocol.

The FDA also conducts audits to confirm that the protocol has been executed correctly, the patients have been consented properly, and all of the data are true. If the FDA has received a complaint about a particular investigator or medical center, an audit could be called for *cause,* that is, the FDA is visiting the site in response to a specific concern. On the other hand, the FDA may choose to do a random audit. Typically, an FDA audit is ordered to review the data when a drug is about to be reviewed for approval. If serious irregularities are found during an audit, the FDA has the authority to suspend all research at the facility. These deficiencies require corrective action before research can continue. If there is evidence of purposeful deception or fraud, the facility could lose the right to conduct any research.

Fraudulent situations are rare, but patients need to be aware of the possibility. All of the safeguards discussed in this chapter are in place for the safety and protection of those who participate in clinical trials. Be certain to determine that the study has been reviewed and approved by an IRB. Know who is sponsoring the study and how patient safety is being monitored. No safety checks can take the place of a well-informed and knowledgeable patient who asks pertinent questions.

■ References

1. Lara PN, Higdon R, Lim N, et al. Prospective evaluation of cancer clinical trial accrual patterns: identifying potential barriers to enrollment. *J Clin Oncol* 2001;19:1728–1733.
2. Dunham W. Cancer patients not keen to be test subjects. Available at *http.www.cnn.com/2001/HEALTH/conditions/03/14/cancer.patients.reut/index.html.* Accessed March 14, 2001.
3. Sinclair U. *The jungle.* New York: Doubleday, Page & Company, 1996.
4. International Conference on Harmonisation. Good clinical practice: consolidated guideline: notice of availability. *Federal Register* 1997;62:90.
5. The Nuremberg Code [from *Trials of War Criminals before the Nuremberg Military Tribunals under Control Council Law No. 10.* Nuremberg, October 1946–April 1949. Washington, DC: US Government Printing Office, 1949–1953].

Available at *http://www.ushmm.org/research/doctors/Nuremberg_Code.htm.* Accessed March 16, 2001.

6. McCarthy CR. Historical background of clinical trials involving women and minorities. *Acad Med* 1994;69:695–698.
7. Consumer protection, where do we stand? World Consumer Rights Day 1999. Available at *http://www.consumersinternational.org/rightsday99/.* Accessed March 16, 2001.
8. National Commission for the Protection of Human Subjects of Biomedical and Behavioral Research. *The Belmont Report.* DHEW Publication No. (OS)78–0013 and (OS)78–0014. Washington, DC: US Government Printing Office, 1978.
9. *Federal Register* 62:90.
10. Federal regulations and guidelines. Code of federal regulations. *Federal Register* 1996;61:192.
11. U.S. Food and Drug Administration Center for Drug Evaluation and Research. Oncology tools. Available at *www.fda.gov/cder/cancer/index.htm.* Accessed March 9, 2001.
12. Mulay M. *Step-by-step guide to clinical trials.* Sudbury, MA: Jones and Bartlett, 2001:23–27.

CHAPTER 8

How to Find a Clinical Trial

■ Locating Clinical Trials

Thousands of clinical trials are conducted all over the world. Locating a trial that fits a specific patient's needs may seem like putting together a jigsaw puzzle.

Primary physicians and local oncologists should be able to help patients locate major cancer centers in their area. They often know an oncologist at a nearby cancer center who can help connect their patients to people who are conducting research. The more common the diagnosis, i.e., lung or breast cancer, the easier it will be to find a clinical trial.

Unfortunately, patients often complain that their doctors are not able to give them information about current clinical trials or how to contact people who do know. There is an information service for physicians, called *Physician Data Queries (PDQ)*, that is sponsored by the National Cancer Institute (NCI). A physician can access it from his or her personal computer or at a medical library and receive the latest information on clinical trials being offered all over the country for every type of cancer. Ask for a search to be done for the patient's diagnosis.

Nonetheless, the onus of locating appropriate clinical trials often becomes the responsibility of the patient or family, and only the most resourceful succeed. This next section will help make that task easier.

National Cancer Institute

The NCI is an arm of the National Institutes of Health in Bethesda, Maryland. The NCI provides the Cancer Information Service (CIS), which can be reached by calling 1-800-4-CANCER (1-800-426-6237). When calling that number, request a customized search of the PDQ database, which will give information on current studies. Also request the pamphlet, *What Are Clinical Trials All About?* It will give more information about the clinical trials and help formulate questions.

The NCI also can be contacted via the Internet. The home page can be accessed at *http://cancernet.nci.nih.gov.* The home page for the NCI's International Cancer Information Center (ICIC) can be accessed at *www.icic.nci.nih.gov.* This web address will provide access to the PDQ database, as well as provide up-to-date information on the prevention, diagnosis, and treatment of cancer.

Although the NCI conducts or oversees many studies, it is not possible for every new drug to be studied there. Some people believe that if a clinical trial is not run by the NCI, it is not legitimate. This is not true. Many important discoveries are made through the cooperation of pharmaceutical companies, academic medical centers, and community hospitals, just to name a few. There are many safeguards in place to ensure the safety and ethics of clinical trials conducted outside of the NCI. This was discussed in Chapter 7.

Cooperative groups, established under the NCI's oversight, conduct clinical trials that test a variety of drugs. The cooperative groups allow physicians working in the community to offer new therapies to patients years before the treatment would otherwise be available. Cooperative groups also allow patients to participate in an NCI trial that is being conducted at a medical center near their home rather than traveling to Maryland, where the NCI is located. In the eastern half of the United States, the group is known as the Eastern Cooperative Oncology Group (ECOG); in the west, it is known as the Southwest Oncology Group (SWOG).

Academic Medical Centers

Academic medical centers all have a physician referral telephone number; many also have a clinical trial's referral line. By calling the main number of the university, patients should be directed to one of those lines. If that is not the case, ask to speak to the director of oncology services or the director of clinical research.

Most academic medical centers have web sites that contain links to the oncology services, as well as listings of available clinical trials. For people new to the Internet, universities often can be found by searching under *www.universityname.com;* in the case of an educational institution, the listing may be *www.universityname.edu.* The listing usually gives the name of the trial and includes pertinent inclusion and exclusion criteria. When looking at a list of trials, note the phase of the trial and the patient population being targeted. Each web site will list a telephone number at the cancer center. Call and speak to the intake coordinator to obtain answers to questions or to be connected to the study coordinator for the specific trial that seems to be appropriate. Coordinators can readily address questions about protocol eligibility and requirements for participation.

Military and Veterans' Hospitals

Many of the military institutions participate in clinical trials. Patients who are eligible to receive care in one of these institutions will be able to locate information on specific trials by contacting the local veterans' facility or the U.S. Veterans' Administration offices in Washington, DC.

American Cancer Society

The American Cancer Society (ACS) is a rich source of information for cancer patients. The ACS can be reached by calling 1-800-227-2345. The 800 number can direct patients to the local ACS office in their area as well as provide well-written information about specific diagnoses. The ACS also will be able to give information about cancer treatment centers in the patients' geographical area.

Patient Advocacy Groups

One of the benefits of the information technology explosion is the ability of patients all over the world to communicate with each other. Many organizations have been established to disseminate information and support to patients with a certain disease. For example, information on breast cancer clinical trials can be located at the National Association of Breast Cancer home page at *www.nabco.org.* The Wellness Community and similar organizations provide a supportive environment for patients and families, and they are good sources for information. Social workers are an important resource to patients and families. Those who work in an oncology setting have a wealth of current information to solve the practical problems associated with a cancer diagnosis (i.e., transportation, housing, wigs). They also conduct support groups and provide individual counseling.

The Internet

Using the Internet to search for information about a specific type of cancer and its treatment will link patients to information about research being done at various institutions. When searching the Internet, enter the diagnosis as the key word and expect to receive hundreds of pieces of information.

There are chat rooms where patients with similar diagnoses share information. People in a chat room may have already accessed information about clinical trials and can help locate trials for a specific diagnosis. Use caution when participating in a chat room, because it can be a source of misinformation. Remember, the patient's doctor is the best resource to discuss information and relate it to a specific situation.

■ Determining Eligibility

Whether clinical trials are located on the Internet or by speaking to an intake person at a cancer center, patients will need to know some basic information about their diagnosis to determine eligibility for a clinical trial. Recall that the inclusion and exclusion criteria of a study define the qualifications. Typically, intake questions include

What is your diagnosis?
Is the disease metastatic?
What treatment have you already received?
When was your last treatment?
What is your significant past medical history?
What medications are you currently taking?

A patient's diagnosis as it appears on the pathology report must match the disease being studied (breast cancer, lung cancer, etc.). Some inclusion criteria also will state the cell type (adenocarcinoma, squamous cell carcinoma, etc.).

If the study is designed for patients with metastatic disease, there must be existing disease that has not been surgically removed. Computerized tomography scans must prove the existence of metastatic disease.

The inclusion criteria for some studies will require a certain number of prior treatments or specific prior treatment(s). For example, a lung cancer study may require that the patient has had only one prior treatment but does not state what drugs were used. Another lung cancer study may require that the patient has had only one prior therapy with carboplatin and paclitaxel (Taxol), the current standard first-line treatment for lung cancer. Some colorectal studies exclude patients who have had more than 25% of their pelvis radiated. Therefore, it is imperative to have records that clearly define the prior treatment (chemotherapy flow sheets, radiation summary). These documents also will give the last date of therapy. Most studies will require that patients have had no chemotherapy for at least 4 weeks before starting the study. Likewise, there typically are parameters for a waiting period between surgery or radiation and starting the study.

Knowing the patient's past medical history will help to define eligibility. These parameters are established because some prior or existing condition or medication may increase the patient's risk when taking the study medication. For example, if there is a history of coronary artery disease and angina (chest pain), a study drug that affects blood flow to a tumor also may affect blood flow to the heart. In people with normal heart function, the drug will have no adverse reaction; however, in people with existing cardiac problems, the drug may cause a heart attack.

Similarly, a drug the patient is currently taking may interact with the study drug. Let us look at this scenario. The study drug is an oral medication. A patient with heartburn is taking a drug to block stomach acid. Changing the acid content of the stomach may change the way the drug is absorbed into the patient's body or change the chemical structure of the drug. In some cases, patients may be able to stop the current medicine, change the schedule to not interfere with the study drug, or switch to a different medicine that will not be a problem. Other times, some medications, such as antiseizure drugs, cannot be changed without placing the patient at undue risk.

Patients must be completely honest about their medical history and current medications when planning to enroll in a clinical trial. Remember that the inclusion and exclusion criteria are established not only to clearly define the patient population, but also to ensure patient safety while the patient is in the study.

If a study is designed to look at patients with metastatic lung cancer and the potential study patient has breast cancer that is metastatic to the lungs, the patient is not eligible. Patients sometimes believe that if breast cancer metastasizes to the lung, they then also have lung cancer. This is not correct. Breast cancer metastatic to the lungs is still breast cancer. Breast cancer metastatic to the bone is not bone cancer.

Exceptions

In some cases, a patient may have a minor deviation from the inclusion and exclusion criteria. A physician may ask the sponsor for an **exception** for this patient to participate. For example, if the total white blood count must be 2.0 to start the study and the patient's white blood cell count is 1.9, the investigator may ask for, and receive, an exception for the patient to enroll. On the other hand, if a drug is known to potentially cause kidney damage, the exclusion criteria will eliminate patients with a creatinine level (a blood test that defines kidney function) over a certain value. Asking for an exception in this case would not be responsible or safe.

The right to grant exceptions lies with the sponsor, not the physician or study coordinator. It is important to remember that the inclusion and exclusion criteria not only define the patient population, but they also establish parameters for safe administration of the study drug. Because patient safety is the primary concern, exceptions are rare and only granted when they will not compromise a patient's safe participation in the study.

If the patient is ineligible for a specific clinical trial, look for another trial. Although a patient with very abnormal laboratory values may not be eligible for any study, large medical centers are likely to have other options for patients who fail to meet the other inclusion criteria. For example, if a particular study excludes patients who are taking antacids, it is likely that there is another study that does not. Because most clinical trials have scientific merit, patients should not agonize over being ineligible for a particular trial.

■ Patient Advocates

Clearly, locating clinical trials can be time consuming and may be too overwhelming for a person who is dealing with the physical and emotional demands of cancer. Therefore, having someone who advocates for the patient in locating available trials may be very useful. It is important that the advocate have all of the pertinent information about the patient's diagnosis and prior treatments in order to accurately identify potential trials. If there is more than one person helping to locate trials for a certain patient, they should talk to each other to avoid duplication of effort.

Once a trial(s) is located, it is preferable for the patient, not the advocate, to call the medical center to discuss eligibility and the specifics of a particular trial. Intake coordinators want to ensure that the patient is truly interested in participation and is not being represented by a well-meaning but overzealous relative or friend.

Patients should keep their primary physician informed of the decision to seek participation in a particular trial. As an ongoing interest in the patient's welfare, the primary physician may need to initiate insurance referrals for participation (see Chapter 9).

A frank discussion between the patient and the treating oncologist is a good means to evaluate the merits of a trial. Maintaining good communication among study personnel, the primary physician, and the treating oncologist is also in the patient's best interest. Ask the study personnel to keep the referring physicians appraised of the patient's progress during the trial.

Understanding the Finances

Who pays the bills? The financial obligations of a patient participating in a clinical trial often are misunderstood. Although the patient's financial responsibilities are described in the informed consent, patients frequently do not pay close attention when reading the section on financial obligations. They mistakenly believe that because the drug company is testing a new drug or combination of drugs, all expenses will be covered. This is not true. Also, patients who are part of a health maintenance organization (HMO) present additional challenges. All issues surrounding financial responsibilities must be discussed carefully, in detail, prior to the patient signing the consent. Who is responsible for what is determined by the specific requirements of the study. Further, a patient's insurance will dictate which expenses will be the responsibility of the patient.

■ Controversy over Costs and Payments

Many insurers exclude coverage for services provided as part of a clinical trial because they are defined as experimental (1). But decisions from insurers typically are made on a case-by-case basis, and the decisions are unpredictable. Public and private efforts are under way to remove insurance barriers to patient enrollment (2).

The costs of participation in clinical trials compared with the costs of standard care are the focus of many studies. One study conducted at the Mayo Clinic compared 61 patients in phase II and III clinical trials with matched patients not enrolled in clinical trials. It showed 10% higher costs incurred by the trial patients over a 5-year period (3). Another study at a large HMO (Kaiser Permanente Northern California) looked at a group of 135 patients enrolled in National Cancer Institute (NCI)-sponsored clinical trials over 1 year. Similarly, those patients had approximately 10% higher costs associated with their care. These higher costs were mostly attributed to the administration of chemotherapy (4).

The good news is that efforts to remove some of the barriers have paid off. The NCI now has agreements with the United States Department of Defense and the Department of Veterans Affairs to provide their beneficiaries with coverage when participating in NCI-sponsored clinical trials. Some states, namely, Virginia, Maryland, Illinois, and Rhode Island, have passed laws mandating at least partial coverage for patients participating in federally approved clinical trials. In June 2000, President William J. Clinton signed an executive order mandating that Medicare cover routine costs associated with clinical trials. This mandate applies only to trials that have therapeutic intent, thereby excluding phase I trials. Nonetheless, this is particularly encouraging, as cancer afflicts so many people over the age of 65 years (5).

Although work is under way to improve insurance coverage, each situation is unique. It is important for each individual anticipating enrollment to understand the costs associated with a specific trial and to be clear about coverage and out-of-pocket expenses.

■ Cost of the Study Drug

When a patient participates in a study of an experimental drug, the cost of the drug as well as all costs of administration of the drug will be paid for by the study sponsor (pharmaceutical company). For example, if a patient enrolls in a phase I study of a new intravenous (IV) drug, the sponsor will provide the drug and pay for its preparation, including the cost of the IV bag and tubing. The cost of the administration of the drug (i.e., the treating nurse and treatment facility costs) also is the responsibility of the sponsor.

The situation becomes more complex if the patient is participating in a study that combines an experimental drug with a United States Food and Drug Administration (FDA)-approved drug. In this case, just as indicated above, the sponsor will pay for all costs associated with the experimental drug. However, the cost of the FDA-approved drug and its administration (preparation, equipment, and administration costs) typically are billed to the patient's insurance company. For example, a patient is enrolled in a study combining experimental drug AB45 with paclitaxel (Taxol), an FDA-approved drug. AB45 is given intravenously over 1 hour and then Taxol is given intravenously over 3 hours. The sponsor provides the AB45 and pays for its preparation and administration, including 1 hour of nursing care and treatment room time. The cost of Taxol, its preparation, and its administration (IV bag, tubing, nursing time, and treatment room time) is billed to the insurance company. The rationale is that the Taxol is a reasonable drug to treat the patient's disease and, therefore, should be covered by the insurance company. If the patient were not participating in this trial, he or she would be receiving some other therapy or Taxol alone, which the insurance company would be expected to cover.

■ Cost of Laboratory Tests

Patients in clinical trials typically have frequent blood tests to ensure their safety while receiving an experimental treatment. The study sponsor pays for some of the blood tests and others are billed to the insurance company.

It is the standard of care that patients receiving chemotherapy have weekly complete blood counts (CBC) to monitor the effects of the drug(s) on their blood cell production. A CBC defines the various components of a patient's blood, such as white blood cells (including several types of white cells), red blood cells, hemoglobin, hematocrit, and platelet count. A weekly CBC while a patient is participating in a clinical trial is billed to the patient's insurance company because it is the standard of care.

On the other hand, a serum chemistry panel typically is drawn monthly for patients receiving chemotherapy. A chemistry panel tests the patient's electrolyte levels, blood sugar, kidney, and liver functions. However, patients participating in some clinical trials, particularly phase I studies, may have a weekly chemistry panel to ensure that the experimental drug is not adversely affecting the body's normal functioning. Therefore, the sponsor will pay for three of every four chemistry panels and one each month will be billed to insurance.

Sometimes, the sponsor may require additional blood or urine tests beyond the standard testing. The need for extra tests often is driven by a toxicity (side effect) seen during the animal studies. For example, in preclinical testing, a drug may have caused an elevation in triglycerides when given at very high doses to the animals. Although the patients are receiving a much lower dose, the sponsor may choose to check a triglyceride level every week to ensure that a similar phenomenon does not occur in humans. The sponsor will pay for any tests that are not considered standard of care and are done specifically to monitor the effects of the drug.

▋ Other Costs

Computerized tomography (CT) scans typically are done every 8 to 12 weeks to monitor a patient's progress while on treatment. Insurance companies consider the 8- to 12-week interval the standard of care. However, a sponsor may require that CT scans be done every 6 weeks to closely track the patient's response to an experimental treatment. In this case, the sponsor will pay for every other set of CT scans. If an experimental drug has the possibility of cardiac toxicity, the sponsor may require a monthly electrocardiogram or other more sophisticated cardiac testing. Because these tests are directly related to the experimental nature of the study, the sponsor has the responsibility to pay for the tests.

▋ Insurance Issues

The costs of health insurance are among the most expensive benefits a company provides to its employees. Employers search for a reasonable insurance plan at the minimum cost. Some larger companies now offer their employees several choices. Plans that allow the employee more choices about their medical care typically have higher premiums.

Some companies offer tiered plans: level 1 is a health maintenance organization (HMO), level 2 is a preferred provider organization (PPO), and level 3 is an indemnity policy. At the HMO level, a patient has a primary physician who acts as a gatekeeper and must either provide all of the patient's care or give referrals to a specialist as he or she deems necessary. A small copayment, typically $5 to $10 per visit, must be paid to see the primary physician or specialist when a referral has been issued. For a larger copayment, patients can choose to see a physician who is a preferred provider within their system. Other systems have a 90/10 payment schedule when using a PPO, meaning the patient must pay 10% of all costs associated with care given under the PPO tier. The indemnity level is even more expensive to the patient, typically an 80/20 system, with the patient paying 20% of all costs billed to insurance.

When a patient with a managed care insurance is contemplating participation in a clinical trial, the insurance company must give authorization to ensure that expenses typically billed to the insurance company will be paid for. The informed consent usually states that the patient is responsible for any costs not covered by the insurance company.

■ Authorizations

It is the patient's responsibility to obtain referrals or authorizations to participate in a clinical trial. Many medical centers have managed care offices to assist in the authorization process by providing insurance companies with necessary documentation. Research teams often write letters to insurance companies to help facilitate authorizations. However, the final responsibility remains with the patient. Without authorization, the patient is expected to pay for all expenses that would otherwise be billed to the insurance company.

Many medical centers refuse to schedule appointments for patients who do not have referrals. Money lost from bad debts has placed many institutions in financial jeopardy. Therefore, if authorizations are required, patients must understand what authorizations are needed, when they must be secured, and who is responsible for obtaining them.

■ Self-Pay

Some patients may choose to pay out of pocket for study-related expenses. This could be a very costly choice. Before making the decision, patients should ask the study coordinator for a clear accounting of all charges. If the study charges include an FDA-approved chemotherapy drug, be prepared for very high costs. Drugs and the cost of administration can be prohibitively expensive. CT scans also are very costly. Even one cycle of therapy could cost several thousand dollars.

■ Housing and Transportation Costs

Patients may choose to participate in a clinical trial that is located in a medical center far from their home. Some studies require that the patient make frequent visits to the medical center, but sponsors rarely pay for housing costs. Sometimes, there is a problem finding temporary housing; when available, often it is very expensive. Other times, patients may choose to travel from home to the medical center for required appointments. Depending on the study requirements, and where the patient lives, he or she could be driving or flying hundreds of miles each week. Patients must consider not only the financial burden of this kind of commitment, but also the time involved.

Depending on the treatment, patients may need someone to drive or accompany them to their treatment appointments. Consideration must be given to the availability of a companion and the potential additional travel expenses.

■ Adding up the Costs

Patients must consider the long-term effects of financial commitments prior to enrollment in a study. Some may feel that the cost of housing for 2 months is an acceptable expense. But if the therapy is successful and the patient continues for a year or more, will the expenses still seem reasonable?

Patients and their families must look realistically at the potential benefit of the treatment versus the costs, both financial and emotional, of participation in a particular study. The decisions often are based on the family's financial situation and their value system. Decisions concerning money must be made as objectively as possible.

■ References

1. US General Accounting Office. NIH clinical trials: various factors affect patient participation. Washington, DC: US General Accounting Office, 1999, Publication no. GAO/HEHS-99-1821.
2. Goldman DP, Shoenbaum ML, Potosky AL, et al. Measuring the incremental cost of clinical cancer research. *J Clin Oncol* 2001;19:105–110.
3. Wagner JL, Alberts SR, Sloan JA, et al. Incremental costs of enrolling cancer patients in clinical trials: a population-based study. *J Natl Cancer Inst* 1999;91:847–853 (published erratum appears in *J Natl Cancer Inst* 2000; 92:164–165).
4. Fireman B, Fehrenbacher L, Gruskin EP, et al. Cost of care for patients in cancer trials. *J Natl Cancer Inst* 2000;92:136–142.
5. Health Care Financing Administration. Medicare coverage policy: clinical trials. Available at *http:www.hcfa.gov/coverage/8d2.htm*. Accessed March 23, 2001.

CHAPTER 10

Care of the Research Subject

Once an appropriate clinical trial has been located and the candidate has undergone preliminary screening with the research staff, he or she is scheduled for an appointment in the investigator's clinic. The final determination of an individual's eligibility for a specific protocol is decided during the **screening visit.**

■ Information Gathering

During the screening visit, a candidate for clinical trial is seen by the research staff to gather all necessary information for participation in the trial. Just like a consultation, a detailed history of the current illness is reviewed. In order to facilitate the process, it is important that complete records are brought to the visit, including

Pathology report
Operative reports
Chemotherapy flow sheets
Radiation summary
Recent computerized tomography (CT) scans and reports
Recent blood work results

The candidate's past medical history, including allergies and current medications, is noted. Typically, the candidate also will be asked questions about family history, such as the occurrence of other cancers in the family. A social history will include questions about smoking and alcohol use, and possible work-related exposures to cancer-causing agents. The candidate will be asked to describe his or her current symptoms, such as fatigue, cough, or nausea. It is important to establish the baseline symptoms to differentiate between current symptoms and possible side effects of the experimental drugs when treatment is started. A physical examination concludes the information-gathering portion of the visit.

■ Presenting Options

Once the information gathering is completed, a physician who is an investigator in the clinical trial will explain the treatment options. Typically, the candidate is advised that there are three options: no treatment, standard treatment, and experimental treatment. Even though the purpose of the visit is to screen for a particular trial, every potential candidate must be told of all available treatment options.

If it is established that the candidate prefers the option of experimental therapy, the investigator will explain all aspects of the particular trial(s) that are appropriate for this patient. A detailed description of how the drug works, the known side effects, and results of previous studies are presented by the investigator. Often the patient has already heard this information from earlier telephone conversations with the research staff. Nonetheless, the investigator must satisfy his or her responsibility to ensure that the candidate has been fully informed. The candidate then is given the opportunity to ask questions.

■ What to Ask

Before going forward with the consenting process, a patient must understand how the specific trial works in general and what he or she can expect in particular. The following questions may serve as a guide:

What is the objective of the study? What does the treatment involve (frequency of visits and time per visit)?
Does treatment involve hospitalization?
What side effects are expected?
How long will the study last?
If the treatment helps, how long can the patient continue?

What are the costs to the patient?

If the patient is harmed by the study treatment, what treatment will be given and who will pay for it?

After the study is over, what is the long-term follow-up care?

Write the questions down to be sure not to forget them. Write or tape record the answers so that they can be referenced at a later time. Many of the questions can be asked during the intake process rather than the screening visit to avoid lengthy consultations for a study that is unacceptable to the patient.

■ The Consenting Process

The candidate may have already read the consent before coming to the screening visit. Even if that is the case, the candidate may be asked to read the informed consent form again and, when all questions have been answered, sign the consent. The candidate may choose to take the consent home and share it with family members or advisors before signing to participate in the trial. It is important that the candidate take as much time as needed to understand fully the requirements of the study. No patient should feel coerced. The informed consent form should include a statement that a decision not to participate in the trial will not adversely affect the patient's care.

Once the candidate decides to participate in the clinical trial, the informed consent must be signed, dated, and timed. The investigator also signs, dates, and times the consent. A copy of the fully executed consent form is given to the candidate, who is now the participant. No trial related testing can be done until the informed consent form has been signed. Because participation in a clinical trial is voluntary, a patient may withdraw consent at any time. However, once a patient has signed a consent, even if consent is withdrawn, the research staff usually is required to continue to follow the patient's progress with periodic telephone calls.

■ Screening Examinations

The purpose of screening is to ensure that the patient meets all eligibility criteria. Although some of the information can be determined over the phone, many protocols demand that the final screening be completed within 7 to 14 days before the patient begins the study drug.

The final screening includes blood tests and a physical examination to determine that the patient does not have any problems that would interfere with his or her participation in the study. Most commonly, a complete blood count is done to ensure that the patient is not severely anemic and has adequate platelet function. A blood chemistry panel is done to check the patient's kidney and liver function, and, when appropriate, a tumor marker is drawn. CT scans are performed to establish a baseline assessment of the extent of the disease.

■ Registration with the Sponsor

If all of the test results fall within the parameters of the eligibility criteria, the patient is registered with the sponsor as a participant in the study. Typically, a screening checklist, which is a list of all inclusion and exclusion criteria, is completed, indicating that the patient satisfies each criterion. A member of the sponsor's clinical staff reviews the checklist, signs it as agreement that the patient is eligible for participation, and telefaxes it back to the investigator. A patient cannot receive the study drug until the completed registration form has been received at the medical center.

■ Randomization

In a phase III study, after a patient is registered with the sponsor, he or she must be randomized to a specific treatment arm. The process of randomization typically is done via telephone into a computerized system. The program prompts the caller to enter specific information and then assigns the patient to one of the treatment arms.

Stratification

Stratification is a system used to ensure that the arms of the study are comparable. For example, the same number of men and women should be on each arm of a study. If the study allows for patients with performance status of 0, 1, and 2, stratification will ensure that all arms include equal numbers of patients at each functional level.

■ Treatment

The treatment schedule is defined by the individual protocol. Even if treatment is every 3 weeks, the study may require that the patient be seen every week. The frequency of visits to the medical center often is dictated by the phase of the study. For example, in a phase I study, because information about the drug is limited, visits may be more frequent than in a phase III study. For safety reasons, a patient must comply with the study schedule. Failure to do so could result in the patient being taken off the study.

Pharmacokinetic Testing

Pharmacokinetic testing is done most often in phase I trials. Recall that one of the objectives of a phase I study is to determine how the drug is metabolized. In order to understand this process, blood is drawn at frequent intervals before, during, and after the patient has taken the study drug. The blood is analyzed through a special process to determine how the drug is broken down and utilized by the body. The amount of time the drug stays in the patient's body (the **half-life**) also helps determine how frequently the drug can be given safely and/or how often it must be given to maintain its effect on the tumor.

Take the example of an intravenous (IV) drug that infuses over 2 hours. Typically, on the first day of treatment, a patient will have a preinfusion PK blood draw, one 30 minutes after the infusion starts and one 90 minutes after the infusion starts. Following the infusion, PK blood draws also may be done every one-half hour to hourly for 3 to 6 hours. The length of time of postinfusion PK draws often is dictated by the length of time the drug stayed in the animals' systems in preclinical testing. Sometimes, a patient may be asked to return the next morning for a 24-hour PK.

If a drug is given intravenously, a second IV line must be started to draw the PK blood at a site away from the infusion site. Therefore, even if a patient has a central venous catheter (Port-a-Cath), another IV line will be started. Treatment nurses typically will cap off the second IV line, which allows frequent blood draws without the need to repeatedly stick the patient.

Reporting Adverse Events

During each visit, the patient will be asked about any symptoms (adverse events) that have occurred since starting to take the study medication. It is important that the patient accurately report all changes. A mild or subtle change can be reported at the next visit. However, if a new symptom is serious or severe, the investigator or coordinator should be notified as soon as possible.

When a new symptom occurs, a study coordinator typically will ask the following questions:

Have you ever experienced this before?
When did it start?
Did you take any medication for the symptom?
When did it stop?

It may be difficult for a patient to recall all of the details about each minor event that occurs. Therefore, it is a good idea for patients to keep a diary to record all of the information.

No matter how insignificant a symptom may seem to an individual patient, it must be reported. In a dose-escalation study, a subtle symptom at a low dose may herald the possibility of a more serious event at a higher dose.

Based on preclinical testing or early human trials, some symptoms or side effects of the drug are expected. However, if a previously unknown but serious side effect occurs that is determined to be related to the study medication, special reports must be filed with the sponsor and the United States Food and Drug Administration. Any hospitalization, even if elective (planned in advance), is called a *serious adverse event* and requires special reporting.

Serious adverse events must be reported to the sponsor within 24 hours of the investigator learning of them. Therefore, if a patient is admitted to a hospital, the investigator should be notified immediately.

Restaging

At prescribed intervals, CT scans are repeated to determine if the study drug has had any effect on the disease. Each protocol defines parameters of response, stable disease, or progressive disease. If the disease has not progressed (grown), a patient may continue to receive the study medication. Scans will be repeated at the next prescribed interval and the patient will continue to receive the study medication as long as it is controlling the disease or until there is no longer any objective evidence of disease.

Termination from the Study

A patient will be removed from a study if the scans show that the disease has progressed. Progressive disease indicates that the study medication is no longer helping.

If a patient experiences a severe side effect, for example, an allergic reaction to the drug, the investigator will remove the patient from the study for safety reasons. Because participation in a clinical trial is voluntary, a patient may withdraw consent at any time.

Follow-Up Requirements

A follow-up visit typically is scheduled 1 month after a patient has terminated from a study. The purpose of the visit is to ensure that any adverse events that occurred during the trial have resolved and no late symptoms have occurred. If any serious adverse event (hospitalization) occurs during that 30-day period, the investigator should be immediately notified.

Many studies require that long-term follow-up be conducted on all study participants. As long as the sponsor continues to collect data on the specific study, study personnel will call the patient approximately every 3 months to determine the patient's status. They usually will ask about additional treatment and/or CT scans the patient underwent since leaving the study.

■ Patient Versus Research Subject

Although a patient's participation in a clinical trial is very important, the study is not more important than the patient, that is, the care of the patient supersedes all study requirements. Therefore, if the patient's medical needs are in conflict with a study requirement, the patient comes first.

For example, during participation in a clinical trial, a patient may develop a painful, cancerous lesion in a bone that requires radiation. The effects of simultaneous treatment of radiation with the study medication may not be known. The need for the radiation is more important than continued participation in the trial, and the patient would be referred for radiation therapy.

The investigator carefully evaluates each situation to determine if the patient's needs and the study requirements are compatible. However, if the circumstances indicate a conflict, the medical needs of the patient win out.

Note that this discussion has been about medical needs. There may be other emotional or social needs that conflict with the study requirements. For example, a patient may wish to take a week or two off of treatment to go on a vacation. Usually, these requests can be accommodated if they are discussed with the investigator in advance. Flexibility in scheduling vacations or other social events to coordinate with study requirements can result in an amicable situation for everyone.

CHAPTER 11

Making the Decision

Many patients assume that their physicians will refer them to a clinical trial if that is an appropriate treatment option. However, a recent study done at the University of California Davis demonstrated quite the contrary. The study looked at 276 patients and found that doctors failed to refer approximately 38% to clinical trials without reviewing their eligibility. The physicians often assumed that there were no appropriate trials or that the patients were ineligible (1).

It is clear that the patient must be his or her own advocate. However, armed with all of the knowledge and options presented in the earlier chapters, many questions may remain.

■ Why Participate in a Clinical Trial?

From a patient's perspective, one advantage of participation in a clinical trial is the possibility of receiving a treatment that is better than known treatments. Recall that all treatments for cancer were tested first in clinical trials and, therefore, patients may receive an effective treatment years before it becomes commercially available.

Patients who receive care in a research facility typically receive first consideration when new protocols become available because they are known to the investigators. Therefore, if one experimental medication is not effective, there may be other experimental therapies that are appropriate for the patient. Cancer researchers often are aware of new protocols that are open or are about to open at other cancer centers and are in a good position to facilitate referral of patients as appropriate.

Another advantage of participating in a clinical trial is that the patients receive extra careful monitoring. Doctor's visits and blood tests often are done more frequently than for patients undergoing a similar, but well-known, treatment.

Many people participate in clinical trials with the hope of finding some answer to prolong or improve their lives. Some also express the desire to contribute to the greater good by helping to find answers to the cancer problem. Whatever the motivation, the brave patients who volunteer for clinical trials make an invaluable contribution to future generations.

■ Why Not Participate in a Clinical Trial?

On the other hand, it is important to understand the risks of participation. Although the experimental treatment has been tested in the laboratory and in animal studies, there is always the possibility of unknown side effects. Animal testing is not always an accurate predictor of how the drug will behave in humans.

Often, participation in a clinical trial requires a greater time commitment than standard therapy because of the frequency of blood tests and doctor's visits (see Chapter 10). There may be costs involved in participation in clinical trials, such as housing and transportation, that would not be necessary if a patient were treated at a local facility. There may be insurance copayments or deductibles that the patient pays by seeking treatment at a facility outside of their covered network (see Chapter 9).

All of these issues must be considered before the decision to participate is made. The final decision belongs to the patient and not well-meaning family members or friends.

■ When to Participate in a Clinical Trial

As discussed earlier, clinical trials are conducted to test every kind of cancer and all aspects (surgery, radiation, chemotherapy) of cancer treatment. Many people think participation in a clinical trial should be limited to those patients who have run out of all other options. This is not true. For example, a newly diagnosed patient may find a phase III clinical trial comparing the current standard of care to a new treatment that has been proven efficacious in an earlier trial. Regardless of which treatment the patient receives, he or she will be receiving a treatment that has been proven to be effective against his or her disease.

On the other hand, it is not prudent to participate in a phase I or II trial if there are effective, known treatment options that the patient has not tried. It is important to understand that *new does not always mean better*. Unless there are medical concerns about the safety of managing side effects, it is always better to be treated with a drug with a proven track record rather than undergoing treatment with an unknown or unproven drug.

The decision about when to participate in a clinical trial may be dependent on the patient's disease, the stage of the disease, treatments already given, and the availability of clinical trials. Take, for example, the following case of William Smith. In Bill's case, he clearly has other better options than to try experimental therapy at this point in his treatment.

■ Case Study A

William Smith, a 57-year-old father of two, was diagnosed with colon cancer with liver metastases in 1998. The colonic mass was removed during surgery, but there were too many liver lesions to remove or treat with ablation. He then received treatment with 5-fluorouracil and leucovorin weekly for over 8 months without growth of the existing liver lesions.

A CT scan done after eight cycles showed the appearance of a new liver lesion signaling that the current treatment was no longer effective. His oncologist recommended irinotecan (Camptosar) as the next best treatment option. Bill was concerned that one of the side effects could be hair loss, and he wanted to explore other options.

In searching the Internet, he read about a phase I study for all advanced solid tumor malignancies using an oral drug that did not seem to have any adverse side effects. When he contacted the cancer center conducting the trial, the intake nurse recommended that Bill take treatment with irinotecan. She told him that a phase I study tries only to establish the safe dose of the drug and he might receive a dose that was too low to be effective. She further explained that even if he received a dose high enough to be effective, it was unknown if the drug actually worked in colon cancer.

Bill then called another cancer center that was conducting a phase II study of an IV drug specifically for colon cancer. Again, it was recommended that Bill consider treatment with irinotecan before trying an experimental therapy. Bill was reminded that a phase II trial is done to determine efficacy. The intake nurse suggested Bill take a treatment with a drug whose efficacy was known before trying something that was yet unproven.

In contrast, consider the following case of Ellen Kosten.

■ Case Study B

Ellen, a 27-year-old school teacher, presented with a lump in her leg. It was biopsied and found to be soft tissue sarcoma. A CT scan showed metastatic disease in her lungs. Metastatic soft tissue sarcoma is a disease with no known effective treatment.

She had surgery to remove the primary lesion in her leg and was sent to a medical oncologist. He advised her that although many different chemotherapeutic agents had been tried in patients with her diagnosis, to date nothing had really shown any significant response. The down side of these treatments is their side effects, which are quite harsh. Her quality of life could be seriously compromised without much hope of any real benefit.

Ellen went to the Internet to search for experimental therapies. She could not find any phase II or III trials being done in soft tissue sarcoma. She did locate a phase I trial designed to enroll patients with all advanced malignancies. In speaking with the intake nurse, she learned that the drug was in the early stages of testing and she was eligible for the trial.

The questions that Ellen needs to ask about the phase I trial include the following:

What is the treatment regimen, IV or oral drug?
How often will she need to come to the medical center?
What toxicities were seen in the animal studies?
What toxicities have been seen in the humans who have already been treated?
Will she be able to increase her dose if higher doses are found to be safe?
If she receives benefit, meaning a reduction in the size of her lung lesions or stable disease, can she continue to receive the drug indefinitely or until she is no longer benefiting from it?

In Ellen's situation, a phase I trial is reasonable because she does not have other good treatment options. However, in Bill's case, there is a United States Food and Drug Administration (FDA)-approved drug with a known response rate that is available to him outside of a clinical trial. A decision to bypass known therapy in lieu of experimental treatment is not a good choice.

■ Randomization

It is important to remember that when consenting to participation in a randomized study, the patient will not have any choice in the treatment arm. It could be that the patient will be randomized to the arm that is the standard of care rather than the new experimental therapy. Ask if cross-over (see Chapter 5) is allowed and at what point that might happen.

Recall that a randomized study may use a placebo in the control arm. Although placebos are not used frequently in oncology clinical trials, it is important to be clear on this point. When considering a study with a placebo control arm, it is important to ask if cross-over is allowed and, if so, when.

■ Thinking Through the Decision

Objective decisions about cancer treatment are extremely difficult to make. Patients often focus on the potential benefit of an experimental therapy when, depending on the phase of the trial, the benefits, if any, may be completely unknown. Sometimes patients are so happy to be eligible for a trial that they ignore the facts surrounding the financial and time commitments.

Before committing to participation in a clinical trial, patients must be sure to understand all aspects of that commitment. Know exactly how often treatments and visits are scheduled. Know exactly what is being billed to insurance and what is being paid by the sponsor. Know exactly what authorizations are needed and who is responsible for getting them.

■ The Final Decision

Do not commit to something, emotionally, financially, or physically, that is impossible. Is participation in the study going to cause undue financial strain by requiring frequent costly trips to the medical center or necessitating a spouse take time off from work?

Does the trial meet the patient's personal goals? Sometimes families or friends are so zealous about a patient's treatment that the patient feels forced to participate in a trial to please others.

Asking for help in making the decision is sometimes a wise thing to do. Careful selection of the advisor(s) is important. If there is a family member or friend whose opinion is valued and trusted, ask for assistance. Nurses and social workers are excellent resources and can serve as good sounding boards. Talking to other patients who have participated in clinical trials or in the specific trial being considered can be helpful. Read the informed consent thoroughly, ask questions, and take the time to consider all aspects of participation. Use common sense in making the decision. Remember: *new does not always mean better.*

■ Reference

1. Lara PN, Higdon R, Lim N, et al. Prospective evaluation of cancer clinical trial accrual patterns: identifying potential barriers to enrollment. *J Clin Oncol* 2001;19:1728–1733.

Internet Resources

U.S. Food and Drug Administration home page
www.fda.gov

FDA Cancer Liaison Program home page
www.fda.gov/oashi/cancer/cancer.html

U.S. Food and Drug Administration Center for Drug Evaluation and Research
www.fda.gov/cder/cancer/index.htm

NCI PDQ Database
www.cancernet.nci.nih.gov/pdq.htm

Cancer Clinical Trials Database
www.cancertrials.nci.nih.gov

Coalition of National Cancer Cooperative Groups, Inc.
www.cancertrialshelp.org

Glossary

Absolute Neutrophil Count Exact number of neutrophils, determined by multiplying the total white blood count by the percentage of neutrophils; generally required to be >1.5 to give a patient chemotherapy

Adjuvant Therapy Treatment given after surgical resection when no objective evidence of remaining disease exists

Adverse Event Any change experienced by a study subject after enrolling in a clinical trial

AE See Adverse Event

ANC See Absolute Neutrophil Count

Aspirate Fluid withdrawn from a mass; cells withdrawn from bone marrow

Audit Careful review of study data, protocol procedures, study conduct, and/or outcomes to verify that the data are correct and that procedures have been carried out properly. Audits for cause are conducted in response to a complaint or concern about a specific investigator or research site.

Baseline Measurements (laboratory results, tumor measurements) taken prior to starting study procedures and used as the basis to determine response to study treatment

Benign Non-cancerous

Best Supportive Care   Treatment of a patient's symptoms without treating the underlying disease

Bidimensional Measurements   Measurements of the height and width of lesions seen on computerized tomography scan

Blinded Study   Randomized study in which neither the research team nor patient knows which treatment the patient is receiving. The purpose is to avoid bias.

Brachytherapy   Radiation delivered inside the body via radioactive beads or pins

Bronchoscopy   Examination of the respiratory tract by placing a lighted tube through the patient's mouth and into the respiratory tract

Carcinogen   Substance that causes cancer

Causality   Relationship between an adverse event and the study drug

Cell Differentiation   The degree of difference of cancerous cells from normal cells; defined as poorly differentiated, moderately differentiated, well-differentiated

Central Venous Catheter   Tube that is surgically placed into a large vein, i.e., Groshong catheter, for the purpose of drawing blood or giving i.v. drugs

Chemotherapy   Chemical compound used to treat a symptom

Clinical Research Coordinator   Health care professional who is responsible for the organization and execution of study activities

Clinical Trial   Research study to test drugs or devices in humans

Cohort   Group; in a phase I clinical trial, a group of patients who are all treated at the same dose level

Co-investigator   Member of the research team who is responsible for conducting the clinical trial in accordance within good clinical practice guidelines and providing for the safety of the study subjects

Contract   Legal document that is executed between the principal investigator and the sponsor defining their agreement on publication rights, financial matters, and delegation or distribution of authority

Control Arm   In a randomized study, the treatment that is not the experimental therapy

Cross-Over   Ability of a patient to change treatment arms after a given period of time on a clinical trial

Data Manager   Member of the research team who is responsible for recording information about the patients

Distant Metastasis   The spread of cancer to sites remote to the site of origin

Dose-Limiting Toxicity   In a phase I study, an adverse event (usually grade 3 or higher) that is defined as unacceptable and therefore stops further dose escalation

Efficacy   Outcome that defines a drug's ability to relieve symptoms or stop the progress of the disease

Evaluable Disease   Disease seen on radiographic study that does not have discrete boundaries and therefore is not measurable

Evaluable Patient   Patient who has satisfied all protocol requirements and whose outcome is recorded in relation to the study objectives

Exception   Deviation from the protocol that is sanctioned by the sponsor

Excipients   A material in which an active ingredient (drug) is incorporated

Excisional Biopsy   Removal of an entire mass

Exclusion Criteria   Parameters that exclude a patient from participation in a clinical trial

External Beam Radiation   Gamma rays delivered to a specific site to achieve death of cells

Fine Needle Aspiration   Fluid or cells that are withdrawn from a suspicious mass via a needle

FNA   See Fine Needle Aspiration

Food and Drug Administration   Branch of the Health and Human Services of the federal government of the United States charged with regulating the sale of food, drugs, and cosmetics in the United States

Fractionation   Division of a total radiation dose into daily doses

GCP   See Good Clinical Practice

Good Clinical Practice   Standard by which clinical trials are designed and conducted to ensure that data are scientifically valid and the rights of patients are protected

Half-Life   Time required for a living tissue or organism to eliminate one-half of the substance that has been introduced into it

Hematologic Malignancy   Cancer manifested by an abnormal growth of certain blood cells

ICH   See International Conference on Harmonisation

Incisional Biopsy   Piece of a mass removed by making an incision in the patient's skin

Inclusion Criteria   Requirements patients must meet to participate in a clinical trial

IND   See Investigational New Drug

Informed Consent   Document that describes all aspects of a clinical trial

Initiation   The first stage of cancer; a mutation in gene transcription

Institutional Review Board   Institution-specific group of medical and nonmedical professionals who review proposed and existing clinical trials to provide for the safety and rights of research subjects

Interim Analysis Examination of the data usually at the midpoint of a study to review safety and/or efficacy and determine if the study should continue

International Conference on Harmonisation Meeting held to define international guidelines for good clinical practice

Intraoperative Procedures done during surgery

Intraperitoneal Within the peritoneal cavity

Intrathecal Within the spinal canal

Intravenous Within a vein

Investigational New Drug Per *21 Code of Federal Regulations 312.2,* a new drug, antibiotic drug, or biologic drug that is used in a clinical investigation

In vitro In glass; referring to studies performed under artificial conditions in the laboratory

In vivo In life; referring to studies done in living organisms

IRB See Institutional Review Board

Invasion An event characterized by cancer cells spreading from the site of origin and into surrounding tissue

Localized Disease confined to the primary site

Malignant Cancerous

Maximum Tolerated Dose Highest dose of a drug that can be given safely to study subjects without unacceptable side effects

Metabolite Compound produced by metabolism of a drug

Metastasis The spread of cancer from the site of origin

Micrometastasis Existence of disease in a part of body that is not detectable radiographically or by palpation

Percutaneous Intravenous Central Catheter Long catheter placed into a patient's vein by nurse

Performance Status Measure of a patient's functioning in relation to activities of daily living

Pharmacokinetics Analysis of serum drug levels to define metabolites and half-life of a drug

Pilot Studies A clinical trial (usually phase I/II or phase II) utilizing a small number of patients to determine a specific objective. If the objective is met, a larger study will typically be pursued to prove the objective with greater statistical significance.

PK See Pharmacokinetics

Placebo Treatment given with no therapeutic intent

Port-a-Cath Central venous catheter that is placed under the patient's skin

Preclinical Studies Testing of the investigational agent in the laboratory and with animals

Principal Investigator Leader of the research team who is responsible for conducting the clinical trial in accordance within good clinical practice guidelines and providing for the safety of the study subjects

Progression   Growth of index lesions by at least 25% over baseline or the presence of a new tumor

Promotion   Second phase in the development of cancer in a cell; the introduction of a carcinogen

Protectant   Drug given to ameliorate the toxic effects of a drug

Protocol   Written statement of the rationale, objectives, and procedure to conduct a clinical trial

Protocol Violation   Deviation from prescribed protocol procedures

Quality-of-Life Questionnaire   Instrument completed by study subjects to define the patient's daily functioning

Radiosensitizer   Drug that makes cells more sensitive to radiation

Randomization   Arbitrary assignment of patients to a specific arm of a study

Regional Spread   Disease that has spread to local tissue or lymph nodes

Research Subject   Person who volunteers to participate in a clinical trial

Restaging   Repeat scanning to determine disease status

SAE   See Serious Adverse Event

Screening   Initial testing of a patient to determine eligibility for clinical trial participation

Screening Visit   A clinic visit that includes the consenting process, a history, physical examination, laboratory and radiographic testing to determine final eligibility for a specific clinical trial

Sensitizer   Drug that increases the effect of another drug or radiation

Serious Adverse Event   Event that results in death, a life-threatening adverse event, inpatient hospitalization, prolongation of existing hospitalization, persistent or significant disability/incapacity, or congenital abnormality

Simulation   Preparation for radiation treatment to define the site of radiation

Solid Tumor Malignancy   Cancer demonstrated by abnormal, discrete mass of cells

Sponsor   Organization that develops the drug, conducts preclinical research, designs the protocol, and funds the clinical research

Staging   Studies to determine extent of disease

Standard Treatment   Current therapy generally accepted by the medical establishment for the treatment of a certain disease

Stratification   A system to ensure that all arms of a study are comparable

Study Arm   Treatment determined by random selection

Study Coordinator   Person at the site who is responsible for the day-to-day operation of a clinical trial

Systemic   Therapy that is given via an oral or intravenous route to treat the entire body

Total Tumor Burden   The sum of the mass of all measurable lesions

Treatment Arm   In a randomized study, the experimental therapy

Tumor Block   Malignant tissue from a biopsy that is embedded in paraffin wax

Tumor *In Situ*   Cancerous cells on the surface of a structure; cancer at its earliest stage

Tumor Marker   Chemical released by certain tumors

Voluntary   Proceeding from one's own will or consent

Washout Period   Period of time between completing the last chemotherapy regimen and beginning experimental therapy

Index